STDs in the United States

Books in the **Contemporary World Issues** series address vital issues in today's society such as genetic engineering, pollution, and biodiversity. Written by professional writers, scholars, and nonacademic experts, these books are authoritative, clearly written, up-to-date, and objective. They provide a good starting point for research by high school and college students, scholars, and general readers as well as by legislators, businesspeople, activists, and others.

Each book, carefully organized and easy to use, contains an overview of the subject, a detailed chronology, biographical sketches, facts and data and/or documents and other primary source material, a forum of authoritative perspective essays, annotated lists of print and nonprint resources, and an index.

Readers of books in the Contemporary World Issues series will find the information they need in order to have a better understanding of the social, political, environmental, and economic issues facing the world today.

STDs in the United States

A REFERENCE HANDBOOK

David E. Newton

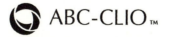

An Imprint of ABC-CLIO, LLC
Santa Barbara, California • Denver, Colorado

Library of Congress Cataloging-in-Publication Data

Names: Newton, David E., author.
Title: STDs in the United States : a reference handbook /
    David E. Newton.
Description: Santa Barbara, California : ABC-CLIO,
    [2018] | Series: Contemporary world issues | Includes
    bibliographical references and index.
Identifiers: LCCN 2017047610 (print) | LCCN 2017048344
    (ebook) | ISBN 9781440858581 (eBook) | ISBN
    9781440858574 (alk. paper)
Subjects: | MESH: Sexually Transmitted Diseases | United States
Classification: LCC RC200.2 (ebook) | LCC RC200.2 (print) |
    NLM WC 140 | DDC 616.95/1—dc23
LC record available at https://lccn.loc.gov/2017047610

ISBN: 978-1-4408-5857-4 (print)
        978-1-4408-5858-1 (ebook)

22 21 20 19 18   1 2 3 4 5

This book is also available as an eBook.

ABC-CLIO
An Imprint of ABC-CLIO, LLC

ABC-CLIO, LLC
130 Cremona Drive, P.O. Box 1911
Santa Barbara, California 93116–1911
www.abc-clio.com

This book is printed on acid-free paper ∞

Manufactured in the United States of America

4 PROFILES, 161

Many excellent books, articles, and web pages contain a host of information about sexually transmitted diseases (STDs; also known as sexually transmitted infections [STIs] or venereal diseases). These resources typically describe the causes of such diseases, the mechanisms by which they are transmitted between individuals, their characteristic signs and symptoms, methods of diagnosis, incidence and prevalence of STDs, and programs for the prevention and treatment of such infections. The literature for young adults is particularly rich in such resources, at least partially because STDs are of such immediate relevance and importance to adolescents. Knowing about STDs is a critical aspect of any young person's personal health perspective.

This book makes no effort to join this extensive list of resources. Instead, it looks at STDs from another perspective, from their role in general society, the way they conform to (or not to) societal norms, their influence on public health, economic complications with which they are associated, political factors that bear on our understanding and treatment of STDs, and other social and cultural issues. The book begins with a somewhat detailed of the history of STDs, going back more than 2,000 years, to times when humans knew little or nothing about the distinction among various types of STDs, let alone their causes or methods of transmission, prevention, and treatment. The story then continues through the 20th century with a review of researchers' ever-improving understanding of the pathogens responsible for such classic diseases as gonorrhea, syphilis, herpes, and hepatitis, an understanding that eventually led to the development of new, targeted treatments capable of acting on these causative agents.

Chapter 2 of the book carries this review into the 21st century when the story of STDs takes some unexpected and crucial variations. After an increasing battle against these diseases in the last decades of the 20th century, epidemiologists are beginning to find that the battle against these classic diseases, along with some new manifestations of sexually transmitted conditions, is not as simple as it might once have seemed. Optimistic assessments for the conquest of syphilis, gonorrhea, and other STDs announced at the end of the 1990s have been replaced in the 2010s by new troubles and concerns: the development of a strain of gonorrhea for which only one drug remains effective, a sudden and unexpected increase in syphilis rates, a continuing explosion in the number of chlamydia cases, a continuing battle against human immunodeficiency virus (HIV) infections, and a debate over the development and use of vaccines against a number of the most common STDs.

STDs in the United States: A Reference Handbook is intended to be just that: a resource on the subject of STDs that will provide a history and background of the topic from ancient history to the present day, with an introduction to the most troubling issues facing the world today. Chapters 1 and 2 are designed to provide readers with the background they need to better understand STD issues, as well as to begin or continue their own research on the topic. Aids for the latter of these objects, further research on STD, are available in Chapters 4 (sketches of important individuals and organizations in STD-related fields), 5 (important data and documents on the subject), 6 (an extensive annotated bibliography of relevant books, articles, and websites dealing with STDs), and 7 (a chronological history of STIs). Chapter 3, called "Perspectives," includes a group of essays by individuals with special interest and expertise in the field of STDs. A glossary of important terms in the field rounds out the book.

This book focuses largely on STD issues in the United States, issues reflected in most developed countries around the world. It does not delve into similar problems and solutions in developing countries, largely because the citizens of those countries generally do not routinely have access to the most advanced forms of prevention and treatment enjoyed by those in developed countries. In addition, the nature of STDs may also be significant in developing, compared to developed, countries. Progress in the battle against HIV/AIDS in the United States, for example, has been hugely successful, while the disease continues to ravage other parts of the world, especially sub-Saharan Africa and parts of the Near East and Asia.

The subject of STIs is one that can present challenges for boys and girls, men and women, of all ages because of the "delicate" nature of the subject. Yet, it is important enough that writers in the field speak clearly about the nature of STDs, which is another objective of this book. A final goal is to provide information that is as up-to-date as possible, given the constraints of producing a print book. Issues related to STDs are often in the daily news, especially in recent years, because of the renewed challenge of dealing with such infections. Understanding such issues and taking a position on them, as may be needed in some circumstances, depends on the availability of such current information.

STDs in the United States

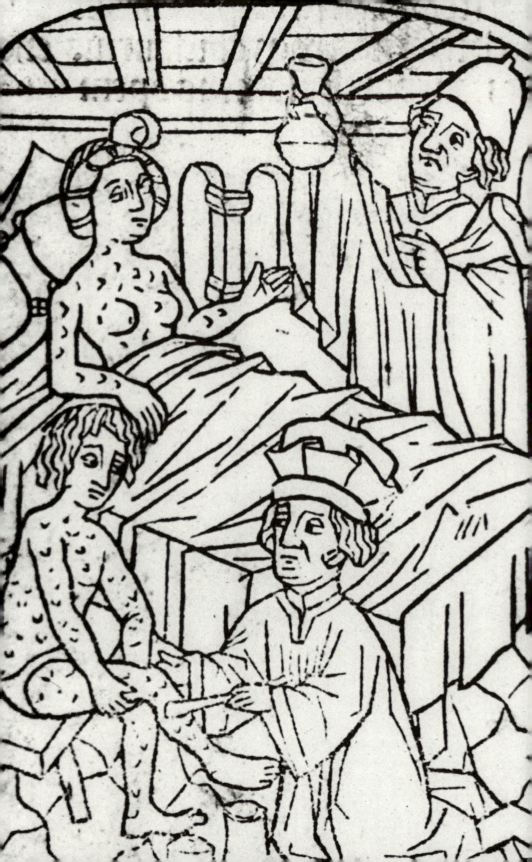

1 Background and History

- Edie: I was so worried when the doctor told me I had chlamydia last year. I guess the one good thing about that news was that I'd never have to worry about having the disease again. Now I'm immune to the chlamydia germ!

- Rodney: Sam and I are so careful about having sex. We never have intercourse, and do only oral sex. That way we can be certain that we'll never get syphilis or gonorrhea or any other sexual disease.

- Andy: I've just had sex with Will for the first time, and I was really careful to make sure he had no signs of sexual disease. I asked him too, and he said he was completely healthy. What a relief!

- Sam: Ginny and I have decided to have safe sex. If I pull out just before I come, neither of us can get a sexual disease. Better safe than sorry!

- Lynette: I'm so glad that I'm taking birth control pills. I know that they protect me not only from becoming pregnant, but also from catching a sexual disease.

Wrong! Wrong! Wrong! Wrong! Wrong!

Many boys and girls, men and women, may think they know all they need to know about sexual diseases to keep themselves

An illustration depicting a woman in bed and a man sitting on a stool, covered with body lesions resulting from venereal disease. A physician stands next to the bed holding up a urine flask for analysis while another physician applies a salve to the man's legs. (National Library of Medicine)

safe. But that may not be the case. All of the above-mentioned statements are wrong; they reflect fairly common beliefs about the way in which sexual diseases can be transmitted from one person to another and what can happen after a person becomes infected. And those misunderstandings are an essential element in the growing rate of sexually transmitted infections (STIs) seen in the United States and many other parts of the world today.

Sexual Diseases

Sexually transmitted diseases (STDs) are conditions passed between two individuals during sexual or genital contact, most commonly through genital, oral, or anal sex. The organisms that cause STDs live in a person's bodily fluids, such as blood, semen, saliva, or vaginal fluids. When a person comes into contact with someone whose bodily fluids contain these organisms, they may also become infected with an STD. STDs were once called venereal diseases, a term derived from the Latin word *venereus*, meaning "sexual love." The Latin word itself comes from the name of the Roman goddess of love, Venus. The term *venereal disease* is not commonly used today.

Another term used for *sexually transmitted disease* is *sexually transmitted infection*. The two terms are almost identical, but not quite the same. The difference arises because a person can become infected with the organism that causes a sexual disease, but may not display any of the outward signs or symptoms of that disease (i.e., be *asymptomatic*). As an example, a common sexual *infection* among women is caused by the human papillomavirus (HPV). HPV infection is a matter of concern because if left untreated it may lead to the development of cervical cancer, a sexual *disease*. So, if a disease-causing organism is present in a person's body, he or she can be diagnosed with an STI. But only if and when visible signs and symptoms begin to appear can he or she be said to have an STD (American Sexual Health Association 2016).

One reason that the term *STI* is becoming more popular today is that some diseases do not show up until many weeks—and sometimes much longer—after a person has become infected. Such is the case, for example, with hepatitis C, a disease that is now considered to be epidemic in the United States. The virus that causes hepatitis C may remain inactive for as long as 10 weeks after an infection has occurred. During that period when a person has no symptoms of the disease, however, he or she may continue to infect other individuals. The use of the term *STI* rather than *STD*, then, helps individuals understand the serious consequences of an infection of which they are not even aware (Boskey 2016).

More than two dozen STIs have been identified. Table 1.1 lists a number of STIs according to the kind of organism that causes the infection, such as a bacterium, virus, or parasite. Some of these infections are quite rare, while others are very common. Basic information about the most common STIs is provided later in this chapter.

Table 1.1 A List of Sexually Transmitted Infections

Cause	Infection
Bacterium	bacterial vaginosis
	chancroid
	chlamydia
	donovanosis
	endemic treponematosis
	genital mycoplasma
	gonorrhea
	lymphogranuloma venereum
	mucopurulent cervicitis
	syphilis
Virus	cytomegalovirus
	Epstein Barr virus
	genital warts
	hepatitis A
	hepatitis B
	hepatitis C
	hepatitis D
	herpes simplex virus (HSV-1 and HSV-2)
	human immunodeficiency virus (HIV)
	human papillomavirus (HPV)
	human T-cell lymphotropic virus (HTLV-1)
	molluscum contagiosum

(continued)

Table 1.1   (Continued)

Cause	Infection
Protozoan	amebiasis
	cryptosporidium
	giardiasis
	trichomoniasis
Parasite	pubic lice
	scabies
	vulvovaginal candidiasis

History of STIs in the Ancient World

Mesopotamia

Historians have long disputed the origins of STIs in human civilization. Some authorities suggest that evidence for the existence of gonorrhea—and perhaps other STIs—can be traced to biblical times and the earliest Mesopotamian civilizations. (One of the best general overviews of the history of STIs from the earliest times through the Middle Ages is Gruber, Lipozenčić, and Kehler 2015.) One report on the presence of STIs in Assyria and Babylonia, for example, argues that existing evidence points to the possibility of at least three forms of STI within these cultures: gonorrhea, chlamydia, and HSV-2 (Scurlock and Andersen 2005, chapter 4). This conclusion is based not only on the symptoms reported on some tablets from the periods involved, but also on current understanding of the nature of sexual interactions that would lead to such problems, such as prostitution. Indeed, the goddess of love in Mesopotamia, Ishtar, was sometimes also mentioned as the goddess of venereal disease (Scurlock 2014, 189). Much depends in this debate on the way in which scholars translate thousands-of-years-old text into modern English. One expert in the field, for example, offers a translation such as this one:

> If his epigastrium [upper abdomen] gives him a burning pain and he is feverish, he eats bread and it does not agree with him, he drinks water and it does not taste good to him and his body is yellow, that person is sick with venereal disease.

If a person's penis and epigastrium hold burning fever,
his liver hurts him and his stomach goes crazy (and) his
arms, his feet, and his stomach are feverish, that person is
sick with venereal disease. (Scurlock 2014, 189; also see
Gruber, Lipozenčić, and Kehler 2015; Paulissian 1991)

A dispute over the presence of STIs during biblical times has
also continued over many generations. An article from 1945 in
the *British Journal of Venereal Disease*, for example, mentions
a number of passages from the Bible that purport to refer to
syphilis or gonorrhea. These include the so-called plague of
Moab (inflicted by God on the Israelites because of their sexual
activity with the women of Moab that resulted in the deaths of
24,000 individuals), the illness that struck Job during the trials imposed on him by God, and the disease that struck King
David as described in the 38th Psalm (Willcox 1949; also see
Burg 2012). Over time, this argument appears to have lost at
least some of its validity, and many scholars seem to agree that
translations of biblical text are too ambiguous to confirm that
STIs were present among people living in the biblical era (see,
for example, Plumb 1997).

Greece and Rome
The status of STIs in ancient Greek and Rome is roughly similar to that described above for earlier civilizations. Greek and
Roman physicians were certainly aware of disorders of the urogenital system, as evidenced by written documents that are still
available today. (The urogenital system in mammals consists
of the organs that make up the urinary and reproductive systems, including the kidneys, ureters, bladder, urethra, testes,
sperm ducts, urethra, penis, ovaries, fallopian tubes, uterus,
and vagina.) One historian, for example, has suggested that
the early Greeks knew of diseases they called "moist ulcers and
phagedenic ulcers," "morbid outgrowths and genital excres-
ences," and "spora," which, the writer argues, correspond to the
modern STIs of genital herpes and chancroid, genital warts,
and scabies, respectively (Morton 1991). He concludes his

review of the place of STIs in ancient Greece with the observation that "the prevalence of both communicable and noncommunicable genital disease was modest" (Morton 1991, 64).

The STI mentioned perhaps most frequently by Greek and Roman physicians was gonorrhea, an STI that one authority has called "one of the oldest known diseases of humans" (Shim 2011). The famous Greek physician, Hippocrates, wrote of a condition that he called *strangury*, with signs and symptoms similar to those of gonorrhea. The disease itself received its modern name from the Roman physician Galen in about 130 CE. Galen conceived of the name—"flow of the seed," in Latin—because he believed that the signs and symptoms of the disease were a result of the release of contaminated semen (Rosebury 1971). Gonorrhea has since antiquity also been known by the name of *the clap*, a term that is thought to have arisen out of its connection with the French name for a brothel, *le clapier* (although other sources are also possible; see Lende 2010). Some evidence suggests that gonorrhea may have existed at least as early as 900 BCE in Japan and may have been prevalent among the ancient Egyptians (Norris 1913, chapter 1).

A number of historians have speculated on the occurrence of other types of STIs among the ancient Romans. Records on the subject are available not only from medical texts of the time, but also from literary sources that deal with health issues of the time. For example, the encyclopedist Gaius Caecilius Pliny (Pliny the Younger) described a malady that he called *profluvium genitalis viris*, a discharge from the penis that might well have been a form of gonorrhea, and ulcers on the genitals that could have been a type of chancroid and perhaps a type of genital warts (Gruber, Lipozenčić, and Kehler 2015, 4). Physicians and other health experts of the time also described a host of medical conditions that might now be characterized as chancroid, genital warts, scabies, nongonococcal urethritis, HPV, congenital syphilis, genital herpes, vulvovaginal candidiasis, and, of course, gonorrhea (Gruber 2015, 4–5; for an example of original text, see Celsus 1935).

Perhaps the most challenging problem in understanding the history of STIs prior to modern times is that of interpreting signs and symptoms reported by writers of the times. For example, Hippocrates described strangury as involving a urinary problem in which urination was difficult and painful, usually resulting in the production of only a few drops of urine at a time, and often accompanied by the appearance of lesions and/or abscesses around the genital organs (Hippocrates 2009). But those signs and symptoms might also be associated with a variety of other renal, nephritic, and urinary diseases other than gonorrhea, with which strangury is often equated by modern observers. And so it is with most of the other descriptions of venereal problems that come down to the modern day from writings from Greece, Rome, and other ancient civilizations, requiring that one use great caution in making observations that are too specific about the status of STIs in the ancient world.

The Middle Ages

For more than a thousand years after the fall of the Roman Empire in 476 CE, little progress was made in the understanding of STIs. During this period, most medical procedures were carried out by individuals with little or no formal training in medicine, such as barber surgeons, apothecaries, and so-called wise women who made use of traditional practices to treat disease. After the founding of the first formal medical schools (Montpellier, 1181; Bologna, about 1200; Oxford, 1220; Perugia, 1321; and Pauda, 1399), more structured training in medicine was available, and the first true physicians became available. But even then, formal medical training and practice remained based on the theories of ancient Greek and Roman physicians, especially Galen. As one observer has written, the driving philosophy in medieval medicine and medical schools was "if Galen figured it all out, why look any further?" (Osborne 2015). Perhaps of equal importance, the reigning philosophy in Europe during this period was the Christian teaching that the world was shortly to come to an end, so that intellectual speculation, such as questions about the nature of STIs, was a frivolous way to spend one's time. As one historian has written, "as God determined the destiny of men, consequently physicians became unnecessary, replaced by prayers and miracles" (Gruber 2015, 6). The diagnosis, theories of etiology, and treatment of STIs during this long period were, therefore, essentially unchanged from the approaches used in ancient Greece and Rome.

One of the interesting changes involving STIs during the Middle Ages was the appearance of laws dealing with its occurrence. Those laws, in turn, were occasioned by an increase in the practice of prostitution throughout most of Europe after about 1100 CE. That change came about as a result of increasing urbanization of the population and a growing need to provide locations for men to satisfy their sexual needs. Many town councils decided that the best way of dealing with this problem was to permit the creation of brothels just outside a municipality's walls where prostitutes could ply their trade. But strict regulations were often adopted to ensure that such establishments were as safe as possible, reducing the likelihood that STIs would be spread throughout the community (Brittain 2015).

The first such law appears to have been adopted in 1162 by the bishop of Winchester in the London suburb of Southwark. That regulation specified that "no stew-holder [brothel owner] to keep any woman that hath the perilous infirmity of burning." A physician of the time explained the meaning of "burning" as "a certain inward heat and excoriation of the urethra, which," he continued, "is a tolerably correct description of the gonorrhea" (Thomson 1812, 174). Similar laws were soon to follow in other parts of Europe, including France and Sicily. In the former case, Louis IX decreed in 1256 that prostitutes with STIs were to be banished, while in the latter, Queen Joanna I ordered that "if one [a prostitute] is found who has contracted a disease from coitus, she shall be separated from the rest and live apart, that she be prevented from conveying the disease to young men" (LaCroix and Putnam 1931; Oriel 1994, 191).

The Appearance of Syphilis

One of the most interesting debates in the history of STIs has to do with the origins of syphilis. That dispute involves at least two distinct theories, the most popular of which are the so-called Columbian theory and the contrasting pre-Columbian theory. According to the former hypothesis, syphilis was brought to the Old World (Europe, in particular) after about 1492 when men sailing on the exploratory voyages to the New World commanded by Christopher Columbus returned home. Along with the news of their discoveries, this theory posits, these sailors carried with them the agents responsible for syphilis, a disease that soon ravaged the continent of Europe. In fact, the first well-documented epidemic of syphilis on the continent dates to about 1494 when an army led by King Charles VIII of France invaded Naples in a war that was to last for four years. At the conclusion of that conflict, the disease had already spread not only throughout Italy, but also well beyond the region covered by the war (Frith 2012).

As a consequence of this sequence of events, one of the earliest names given to syphilis, especially by the Italians, was *morbus Gallicus*, or the French disease. The French, in turn, called the infection *le maladie neapolitan*, or the Italian disease. As the disease spread to other countries, the practice of blaming other countries for its appearance continued, with the French also accusing the Spanish for its rise (*le maladie espagnole*), the Germans calling it *das Französisch Übel* (the French evil), the Russians blaming the Poles (*polirovaniye bolezn*; the Polish disease), the Turks placing the blame on Christians (*Hiristiyan hastaligi*; the Christian disease), the Tahitians called it *the British disease*, the Japanese using the phrase *chugoku no pokkusu* (the Chinese pox), and so on (Frith 2012). The so-called French disease also became widely known at the time, and ever since, as the Great Pox or, much less commonly, the French Pox, terms used to distinguish syphilis from the widespread and greatly feared smallpox (Arrizabalaga, Henderson, and French 1997).

The close chronological relationship between the return of Columbus's ships (1493 for the first voyage) and the outbreak of the syphilis epidemic (1494 or 1495) provides the basis for the Columbian theory of the origin of syphilis. Almost from the moment that the first epidemic broke out, however, other scholars have been arguing for a very different scenario, one in which syphilis had existed in Europe for centuries before the Columbian voyages of discovery. According to this theory, sufficient evidence is available from paleopathology (the study of ancient diseases) to confirm a long-term existence of syphilis in Europe even though written documents of the time may not adequately describe and define the disease. (See, for example, Pàlfi et al. 1992, especially references in the article to other studies.)

Today, the evidence appears to have shifted quite strongly to the pre-Columbian hypothesis for the origin of syphilis. One factor in this change has been the realization that the vast majority of the evidence provided by pre-Columbian researchers has focused on a small number of specific examples in which a diagnosis of syphilis can be as easily explained by some other disease factor(s). More convincing, however, have been a series of genetic studies that trace the presence of syphilis and related diseases (treponematoses), such as bejel, pinta, and yaws. (For a detailed discussion of this research, see Harper et al. 2008; Rothschild 2005.)

According to these studies, a form of syphilis probably first appeared in Africa in either humans or other primates. The disease then spread through Africa, into Asia, and then into the New World. The disease probably reached the New World about 8,000 years ago, and was certainly present when Columbus made his first voyages (Rothschild 2005). This evidence appears to be strong enough that at least one popular scientific journal has announced that the case for the origin of syphilis is now probably closed, and the Columbian theory has won out (Choi 2011). The same article takes note of the social, political, environmental, and other factors that surrounded the spread of syphilis in the 15th and succeeding centuries, as well as the lessons that modern societies can take from this story for the spread of disease in today's world.

Treatments for STIs in History

Whatever ideas medical practitioners may have had about the causes and nature of STIs prior to the Renaissance, one issue with which they inevitably had to deal was the treatment of such conditions. If a person from ancient Egypt, the Roman Empire, or medieval France came to a healer with the symptoms of an STI, that healer would be expected to take some form of action to relieve the pain and suffering of the disease.

The variety of treatments recommended for STIs is considerable, reflecting the almost complete lack of accurate understanding of the source and etiology of these diseases. One history of STIs in antiquity lists treatments such as cold baths; massages; sedatives such as henbane, lentils, lettuce, poppies, and roses; sleeping on a cool bed with a metal plate covering the infected area; ingestion of hemlock; injections of human milk to which have been added almond juice, sugar, and violet oil; and cleansing of the penis with vinegar and water (Norris 1913, chapter 1). Another history of STIs in antiquity mentions the use of a variety of herbs, sometimes soaked into wool tampons for treating the genital region; infusions of sandal oil and other materials; massage with chicory; washing of infected regions with milk and honey; use of aloe dust or the bark of pine trees; application of Spanish fly, leeches, lice, or fleas to the infected area; surgical removal of lesions; and introduction of goat or human milk into the penis or vagina (Gruber, Lipozenčić, and Kehler 2015; also see Rosenbaum 1901).

For syphilis, the two most common treatments were an herb known as guaiacum, or holy wood, and mercury. Guaiacum appealed to healers largely for philosophical reasons; the plant came originally from Hispaniola (Haiti) and was deemed likely to be effective against syphilis, which also was thought to have originated in the New World. Poultices, ointments, tinctures, and other preparations of the herb were used on sores directly, or as preventatives for the disease. The herb was soon found not to be effective either in treating or in preventing syphilis, and healers turned instead to the liquid metal mercury and its compounds. Again, the metal was prepared and used in a variety of ways, most of which were designed to produce salivation and sweating, with the hope that these responses would force the disease out of a person's body. The treatment had some rather serious consequences, however, since many forms of mercury are themselves toxic, causing a range of side effects including loss of teeth; ulcerations of the mouth, throat, and skin; nerve damage; and even death. So a person suffering from syphilis often had the choice of accepting and living with the rather horrible consequences of that disease or submitting to treatments with mercy, which had their own unpleasant consequences, often including death (Treatment of Syphilis in Early Modern Europe 2017).

Any discussion of the treatment of STIs during the medieval period cannot ignore the important role played by religious views on those diseases. These views were based on a belief that the end of the world was near at hand, and Christians should focus on those activities that were likely to bring them eternal life (such as prayers, penance, and observance of rituals), rather than sectarian studies. It was obvious to most theologians that the causes of diseases such as STIs were the actions of supernatural forces, such as works of the Devil, and that the most effective means for dealing with these forces was through religious rituals. This approach to the treatment of STIs was hardly new, but one that can be traced to the earliest days of ancient civilizations. It is perhaps significant only in that it reversed a trend among the ancient Greeks to look for material causes and explanations for physical phenomena, including disease and illness (see, for example, Schlagel 2010; Tarnas 2011). Beliefs in religious treatments for STIs have not completely disappeared from the modern world (see, for example, Healing Prayer for

Sexually Transmitted Diseases, Herpes, Syphilis and AIDS John Mellor Healing 2015; Prayer for Healing of any Diseases and Sickness 2017).

We know very little about the efficacy of these treatments for STIs. One reason for such a statement is the general lack of accurate information among ancient and medieval healers about the course of various types of STIs in general. For example, we know today that a person infected with gonorrhea presents with certain clear-cut symptoms, such as burning during urination and a white, yellow, or greenish discharge from the penis. Early healers would have been able to recognize these symptoms rather easily.

But today's medical workers have further information unavailable to early healers, namely that untreated cases of gonorrhea may have deleterious effects on women in general, pregnant women, newborn children, and infected men. These complications may include a wide variety of conditions, including pelvic inflammatory disease, infertility, chronic and pelvic pain in women in general; preterm labor, premature rupture of membranes, and premature delivery in pregnant women; conjunctivitis, sepsis, and arthritis in newborn children; and infertility in men (Gonorrhea—What Happens? 2017). The problem for early physicians, however, was that few or none of these complications would have been associated with a gonorrheal (or other type of STI) infection. So one could not say whether a treatment for a gonorrheal-like infection was effective or not, because the infection usually just went away on its own, with complications such as these showing up only many years or decades later.

Treatments for syphilis were a somewhat different matter. In the first place, early healers were divided into two camps as to the differences and/or similarities of gonorrhea and syphilis. The "unitarians" believed that the two diseases were actually the same, with one evolving out of the other. One of the most famous proponents of this theory was the famous English physician John Hunter who reputedly (but possibly incorrectly) is said to have inoculated himself with the pus from syphilis lesions, only to develop gonorrhea (Moore 2009). Unitarians believed that mercury was, therefore, the treatment of choice for both gonorrheal and syphilitic infections. On the other hand, the "dualists" were convinced that gonorrhea and syphilis were two entirely different diseases and required two different kinds of treatment.

The dispute between these two schools of thought was finally resolved in 1858 through an elegant series of experiments by the American-born French physician Philippe Ricord. Ricord determined that the progress of a syphilitic infection was distinctly different from that of a gonorrheal infection and that the former could be subdivided into a series of stages well known to any physician today (Pashkov and Betekhtin 2014; Ricord 1842). The first (*primary*) stage in that sequence of events involves the appearance of a chancre (sore) at the point of infection, such as the penis, mouth, or vagina. That stage typically lasts from three to six weeks, after which the chancre disappears and is replaced by a rough, reddish rash that develops around the mouth, the genital region, or on other parts of the body (the *secondary* stage). Once again, these symptoms eventually disappear, sometimes for as long as a year or more later (often called the *latent* stage). At that point, the *final* (or *tertiary*) stage develops, one characterized by damage to many parts of the body, including the brain, nerves, eyes, heart, blood vessels, liver, bones, and joints (Chandrasekar 2016).

The horrors of late-stage syphilis are now well known and widely documented. Again, it may be understandable that early healers did not fully understand the relationship of the three stages of the disease. In any case, as noted above, only one treatment proved to be of any value at all: mercury. And the problem with that treatment was that it was often at least as dangerous and harmful, if not more so, as the disease itself. The medical literature of the ancient world and medieval period is replete with tales of the horrible consequences resulting from treating syphilis with mercury. It is easy to say for this extended period of time, then, that, in many cases, the treatment was a success, but the patient died (see, for example, McDonnell 1881).

STIs: What and How?

By the end of the 16th century, physicians and other healers were relatively familiar with the nature of STIs. They could look at a person with herpes, syphilis, gonorrhea, or some other STI and recognized the condition—by whatever name they might choose to call it—and been aware of possible treatments for the disease, effective or not, as the case might be. The two fundamental things they did *not* know about the diseases were (1) what caused the disease and (2) how it was transmitted from person to person (if they even believed that it was, in fact, a contagious condition). (*Contagious* means capable of being transmitted from one person to another.)

Theories of Miasma

Theories of the "what" and "how" of STIs had been proposed for many centuries prior to the appearance of syphilis in Europe. One of the oldest such theories posited the existence of poisonous vapors called *miasmas* released from swamps, garbage dumps, decaying organic matter, and other sources of foul-smelling air. Theories of miasma can be traced at least to the days of ancient Greece, and probably to much earlier periods of human history. Those theories differed from each other in details, such as to the constitution of miasma itself, but agreed in general that exposure to such vapors was the probable cause of most cases of STIs. One of the first clear descriptions of miasmatic theory was offered by Fracastoro in his 1546 book, *De Contagion*, in which he attributed the occurrence of syphilis in particular to exposure to miasma (Karamanou et al. 2012; Nutton 1983).

Today, theories of miasma are of historical interest only. The explanation for contagious disease that superseded miasmatic beliefs came into being only after a series of discoveries that occurred over a period of nearly two centuries.

Cell Theory to Germ Theory

Our modern understanding of the cause of STIs and many other diseases is based on the *germ theory*, an explanatory system that dates to at least the days of ancient Greece and Rome. The notion that there existed tiny creatures that caused disease and that could be transferred from one person to another was rare during this period, but not entirely unknown. For example, the Roman scholar Marcus Terentius Varro (116 BC–27 BC) postulated a possible germ-like cause of disease in his most famous work, *Rerum rusticarum libri III* (*Agricultural Topics in Three Books*) when he wrote

> If you are forced to build on the bank of a river . . . precautions must also be taken in the neighborhood of swamps . . . because there are bred certain minute creatures that cannot be seen by the eyes, which float in the air and enter the body through the mouth and nose and there cause serious diseases. (Varro 1934, 209)

A more complete and more widely known theory was that of the Italian scholar Girolamo Fracastoro, who, in his 1546 book *De Contagione* (*On Contagion*) suggested that infectious diseases were caused by *seminaria*, or "seeds of disease." Fracastoro thought that these "seeds" could be transmitted from one person to another in one of three ways: by direct contact between an infected and a healthy person; by "indirect" contact, such as by way of clothing or shared utensils; and "at a distance," as in being carried by the wind from infected to healthy individuals. The "seeds" then entered a healthy person's bloodstream, began to decay, and brought on a disease (Echeverria 2010; Nutton 1990).

Theories such as those of Varro and Fracastoro could not be verified, of course, because no mechanism was available to detect and/or study "creatures" or "seeds" that were invisible to the naked eye. The possibility that such agents of disease might exist had to wait until the invention of a device for observing such tiny objects: the microscope. Simple lenses for magnifying very small objectives had been known at least since the ancient Greeks. But the first true compound microscopes, consisting of two lenses that greatly increased magnifying power, did not appear until the work of Dutch inventor Cornelis Drebbel in the 1620s. Devices like those made by Drebbel and, later, by the more famous inventor Dutch inventor Anton van Leeuwenhoek then made it possible for the detection of individual cells (Robert Hooke, 1665) and tiny living organisms (van Leeuwenhoek, 1673; Bardell 2004).

Yet, more than a century and a half were to pass before scholars began to recognize the basic role played by the tiny structures first seen by Hooke, van Leeuwenhoek, and their colleagues. Finally, in 1838, German botanist Matthias Jakob Schleiden formally announced a theory whose existence had long been suspected, namely that all plants are made of cells that are essentially similar to the structures first reported by Hooke 173 years earlier. Only a year later, German physiologist Theodor Schwann extended Schleiden's theory to animals, suggesting that they, too, consisted essentially of a collection of tiny cells. The model was completed in 1845 when German zoologist Karl Theodor Ernst von Siebold suggested that the tiniest organisms then known, such as amoebae and formanifera, actually consist of a single cell. (He also incorrectly hypothesized that more complex, multicellular, organisms were actually made of large collections of these single celled organisms.) The notion that all living organisms of all possible types consist of individual cells—the cell theory—had thus been formulated.

It was a short step from the acceptance of the cell theory to its cousin, the germ theory, the understanding of the nature of infectious organisms ("germs") and the way they cause disease such as STIs. Indeed, some early pioneers had already expressed some thoughts on this concept. In 1720, for example, English naturalist Richard Bradley put forth the notion that very tiny insect-like organisms—too small to be seen with the naked eye—might be responsible for certain types of contagious diseases. He wrote that "all pestilential distempers, whether in animals or plants, are occasioned by poisonous insects conveyed from place to place by the air." Well trained in the use of van Leeuwenhoek's microscopes, Bradley noted that these "insects" would be visible only with such instruments (Bradley 1721; Sanger 2007). (Bradley's work and hypotheses were largely ignored for more than a century.)

In the decades following the work of Schleiden, Schwann, and Siebold, evidence began to accumulate in support of the germ theory, especially the research of the Italian entomologist Agostino Bassi, Hungarian obstetrician Ignaz Semmelweis, English physician John Snow, German physician Rudolf Virchow, and English surgeon Joseph Lister. One of the crucial experiments conducted during the period was carried out in the early 1860s by French chemist and bacteriologist Louis Pasteur. At the time of this research, researchers were still debating the cause of disease, with the theory of miasma holding something of a prominence over any type of germ theory. Pasteur provided conclusive evidence that disease is caused not by vapors in the air caused by decaying organic material, but by tiny microorganisms that exist within a body. The significance of this discovery is reflected in the fact that Pasteur has since often been called the Father of Germ Theory, and his experiments has been described by one of the leading historians of science, Isaac Asimov, as "the greatest single medical discovery of all time" (Asimov 1982, 423).

Of probably equal significance was another series of experiments conducted by German bacteriologist Robert Koch in the decade following Pasteur's discoveries. The first of Koch's discoveries was perhaps the most important, namely that any given disease is caused by some specific microorganism (commonly described as a germ, pathogen, microbe, infectious agent, or causative agent). Koch's work was motivated by an effort to discover the cause of anthrax. Anthrax is a rare infectious disease that occurs naturally in wild and domestic hoofed animals, such as cattle, sheep, goats, and camels, as well as in humans who have been exposed to the infected animals or animal hides. Koch found that a bacterium called *Bacillus anthracis* existed in and could be extracted from animals infected with anthrax. He also found that, when injected into healthy animals, such as laboratory rats, those animals also developed the disease.

In addition to this very specific and important discovery, Koch laid out a series of four "postulates" that could be used to identify the causative agent of a disease. Those postulates (although later found to be somewhat insufficient or inaccurate) were as follows:

- The same organism must be present in every case of the disease.
- The organism must be isolated from the diseased host and grown in pure culture.
- The isolate must cause the disease when inoculated into a healthy, susceptible animal.
- The organism must be reisolated from the inoculated, diseased animal (Grimes 2006, 225).

The Discovery of Causative Agents for STIs

The work of Pasteur, Koch, and their colleagues opened up a whole new field of research for scientists interested in STIs. It was now generally recognized that diseases such as gonorrhea and syphilis were caused by very specific organisms that could eventually be identified, isolated, and studied in detail. Once this information was available, work could begin on the search for specific agents that could kill these agents and cure a disease, without also producing unacceptable side effects.

The first causative agent for an STI was actually discovered well before the work of Pasteur and Koch. In 1836, French physician Alfred François Donné submitted a paper to the French Academy of Sciences entitled "Animalcules observés dans la matière purulente et leproduit des secretions des organs génitaux de l'homme et de lafemme" ("Animalculi observed in purulent fluids and secretions of genital organs from Men and Women"). The disease studied and described by Donné is one now known as trichomoniasis, an infection of the genital region that affects both men and women, but is much more common in the latter than in the former. The Centers for Disease Control and Prevention (CDC) estimates that about 3.7 million people in the United States contract trichomoniasis every year, although only 30 percent experience any symptoms or signs of the disease. Donné eventually named the causative agent *Trichomonas vaginalis* (Diamantis, Magiorkinis, and Androutsos 2009; Thorburn 1974).

The next breakthrough in the identification of causative agents among STIs occurred in 1889 when Italian dermatologist Augusto Ducrey confirmed that a gram-negative bacillus (a disease-causing bacterium), later named *Haemophilus ducreyi*, was responsible for the STI known as *chancroid*. At the time, the disease was more widely known as *soft chancre* (or *ulcus molle*) to distinguish it from syphilis, commonly referred to as *hard chancre*. The two terms refer to the presence of a painless ulcer that appears at the site of an STI, usually the genital region. The ulcer is typically firm and hard in the case of syphilis, and soft in the case of chancroid.

Ducrey was able to confirm his findings by the process of autoinoculation, in which purulent material (pus) taken from a person's genital chancre was injected into his or her arm. As a result of that procedure, a new chancre began to grow on the arm, indicating that the causative agent present in the pus was indeed the cause of the infection. A similar procedure used with the pus from a syphilitic chancre produced no new lesion on the arm, however, also proving that soft chancre was different from hard chancre (Albritton 1989).

Chancroid has always been a rather uncommon disease in the United States, increasingly so in recent years. The CDC reported an incidence of 3,384 cases of the disease in 1941 (2.5 cases per 100,000 Americans). That number increased to 9,515 cases (6.7 cases per 100,000) in 1947, and then began to fall off significantly. According to the most recent data available, there were only 11 cases of chancroid reported in the United States in 2015 (CDC 2016f). Although poorly studied in most parts of the world, statistics for the incidence of chancroid in other developed countries appear to be similar to those in the United States (Mardh, Abrahamsson, and Amato-Gauci 2016).

Possibly the two most important developments following elucidation of the germ theory were the discoveries of the causative agents for gonorrhea and syphilis, long the most serious and widespread of STIs. The gonorrhea discovery was made in 1879 by German physician and medical researcher Albert Ludwig Sigesmund Neisser. Neisser became interested in infectious diseases early in his medical career and went on to become famous for two historic accomplishments—identifying the causative agents of both gonorrhea and leprosy (now known as Hansen's disease)—as well as a number of important and controversial scientific activities. His research on gonorrhea involved the analysis of a new microorganism found in the infected tissue obtained from 26 patients with classical gonorrheal urethritis, as well as 7 cases of neonatal gonorrhea and 2 cases of adult opthalmia, the three most common forms of gonorrhea. All of the samples studied by Neisser contained the same bacterium, a gram-negative gonococcus that was later named in his honor *Neisseria gonorrhoeae* (Benedek n.d.).

Given his successes with the discovery of the Hansen's and gonorrheal causative agents, Neisser launched an effort to resolve the same problem for syphilis. For a number of years, he explored a variety of ways of determining the cause of the disease, discovering precisely how it was transmitted, and identifying ways in which it could be prevented and treated. His passion for unraveling this puzzle led to some experiments that have since been described as examples of unethical human experimentation. In one series of experiments, for example, he inoculated a group of disease-free individuals, most of whom were prostitutes, with fluid taken from syphilitic patients to see if the process would prevent the subjects from developing the disease. The subjects of the experiment were neither informed of the research in which they were involved nor given an opportunity to choose to participate or not (Benedek 2014; Vollmann and Winau 1996).

The ages-long search for a causative agent of syphilis finally reached its conclusion in a series of experiments conducted at the University of Berlin beginning in 1905. (For a detailed history of this search, then in process, see Fanoni 1905.) These experiments were inspired by the discovery of a possible causative agent found in the fluid taken from lesions in patients with primary syphilis by John Siegel, an assistant in the Institute of Zoology at the university. Siegel classified the new microorganism as a type of flagellated protozoan, which he called *Cytorrhyctes luis*. Siegel's discovery was ambiguous, however, because he had found the same protozoan in a number of other infectious diseases, including varicella, hand-foot-and-mouth disease, and scarlatin (thus violating one of Koch's postulates; Macedo de Souza 2005).

Largely ignored by the research community in general, Siegel's discovery prompted the director of the German Imperial Health Institute to initiate further investigations on the role of the flagellated protozoan in the transmission of syphilis. Within a short period of time, the two researchers primarily responsible for this line of investigation, zoologist Fritz Schaudinn and dermatologist Erich Hoffmann, isolated a new microorganism, similar to Siegel's *C. luis* which they unequivocally identified as the causative agent for syphilis. (*C. luis* was not, as it turned out, an organism at all, but organic debris contaminating Siegel's sample.) The organism was described as a spiral-shaped bacterium of the order Spirochaetales, about 5–20 microns in length and 0.5 micron in diameter. It moves rather freely in dilute solutions, but is quite fragile and easily destroyed when not embedded in its host (Rao 2017, slides 13 and 14).

Originally named by Schaudinn and Hoffmann *Spirochæta pallidum* ("white" organism with a "turning head"), the organism was soon given its modern name of *Treponema pallidum*. Before long, confirmatory experiments began to appear in the literature confirming its presence in lesions taken from both primary and secondary stages of the disease. And the final piece of the puzzle was produced in 1913 when Japanese bacteriologist Hideyo Noguchi conclusively demonstrated that the mental disorders (paresis) associated with third-stage syphilis are also associated with *T. pallidum* (Noguchi and Moore 1913). The discovery of *T. pallidum* is a much studied topic in the history of science. Among the best resources on the subject are Oriel (1994, 72–75) and White and Avery (1909).

Two other discoveries of STIs are worthy of note. The first involves the causative agent for a condition now known as vulvovaginal candidiasis (VC). VC is an infection that causes itchiness and burning of the genital region. It is a very common condition that occurs when organisms (yeasts) that occur naturally on the human body grow more abundantly than normal. By some estimates, VC occurs among anywhere between 10 and 30 women per 100,000 in the United States, although these numbers vary widely from location to location. In most cases, VC infections are easily treated and readily cured, although the infection probably never goes entirely away since the causative agent is a natural part of the human body. VC today is not generally regarded as an STI because it can be (and usually is) transmitted by mechanisms other than sexual contact, although intercourse is one possible means of transmission. The general term used to describe all VC-like infections is *candidiasis*, named after the pathogen that causes the disease (CDC 2016b; Vaginal Yeast Infections 2015).

The interesting point for this discussion is that a form of candidiasis also occurs in the mouth, in which case the infection is known as *thrush* (or *oral candidiasis*). Going back at least to the ancient Greeks, thrush was a well-known medical problem because of the discomfort and complications with which it was associated. During the 18th and 19th centuries, the condition occurred most commonly among children and those confined to medical facilities, where conditions were favorable for growth of the organism (Obladen 2012).

The causative agent for thrush was identified almost simultaneously between 1839 and 1844 by three different researchers: Swedish physician Frederik Theodor Berg, Serbian physician David Gruby, and Scottish physician John Hughes Bennett. The person most generally recognized as the organism's discoverer, however, was French biologist Charles Phillipe Robin, who named it *Oidium albicans*. Other names were used until 1923, when it was given its current name of *Candida albicans* by Dutch mycologist Christine Marie Berkhout (Barnett 2008).

The other important breakthrough came only two years after the discovery of the causative agent for syphilis. In 1907, Bohemian zoologist Stanislaus Josef Mathias von Prowazek and his colleague German dermatologist Ludwig Halberstädter reported the isolation of a gram-negative bacterium in the scrapings taken from the infected eyes of orangutans that had been intentionally contaminated with the fluid taken from humans with conjunctivitis. The researchers originally thought that these "inclusions" were protozoans, an error that was later corrected, and the agent was eventually given its modern name of *Chlamydia trachomatis* (the "cloak of blindness"; Black 2013, 1–3).

C. trachomatis is responsible for a number of STIs and other types of diseases, including lymphogranuloma venereum, nongonococcal urethritis, pelvic inflammatory disease, mycoplasma genitalium, trichomoniasis, chlamydial infections, cervicitis, urethritis, prepubertal vaginitis, proctitis, proctocolitis, enteritis, and acute epididymitis (Sexually Transmitted Diseases Treatment Guidelines, 2015). The organism also causes trachoma, an infectious eye disease that is currently the number one cause of preventable blindness in the world (International Trachoma Initiative 2015). Chlamydial infections are also the second most common type of STIs in the United States (after pelvic inflammatory disease). The number of cases of chlamydial infections has risen from 7,594 in 1984 (the first year in which they were a reportable STI in the United States) to 1,526,658 in 2015, the last year for which data are available (CDC 2016d).

The Viral Infections

This review by no means covers the discovery of causative agents for all known STIs. Indeed, of the eight most common STIs in the United States (Table 1.2), half of all causative agents were determined only in relatively recent times. And, in every instance, those agents have been viruses, long among of the most puzzling microorganisms with which diseases specialists have to work.

Although the modern science of virology dates only to the end of the 19th century, viral diseases were known much earlier, even though scholars had essentially no understanding as to the cause of such diseases and the mechanisms by which they were transmitted. Hippocrates is often credited, for example, with the earliest known description of a viral STI, herpes. Indeed, the name itself comes from the Greek word for "to

Table 1.2   Eight Most Common STIs in the United States

STI	Causative Agent	Incidence	Prevalence
HPV	Human papillomavirus	14,100,000	79,100,000
Chlamydia	Chlamydia trachomatis	2,860,000	24,100,000
Trichomoniasis	Trichomonas vaginalis	1,090,000	3,710,000
Gonorrhea	Neisseria gonorrhoeae	820,000	1,570,000
HSV-2	Herpes simplex virus-2	776,000	908,000
Syphilis	Treponema pallidum	55,400	422,000
HIV	Human immunodeficiency virus	41,400	270,000
Hepatitis B	Hepatitis B virus	19,000	117,000

Source: "Incidence, Prevalence, and Cost of Sexually Transmitted Infections in the United States." 2013. https://www.cdc.gov/std/stats/sti-estimates-fact-sheet-feb-2013.pdf. Accessed on February 19, 2017.

creep," *herpein* (Roizman and Whitley 2001). That nomenclature reflects perhaps the most characteristic feature of herpetic infections, itchy or burning blisters or open sores that spread across the lips and mouth or the genital region, that eventually scab over. The infection typically heals without treatment in two to four weeks, although the virus that causes the disease may remain in the body, causing recurrences of the infection at later times (Ayoade 2017). Today, one form of herpes, HSV-2, is the fifth most common STI in the United States, resulting in 299,000 visits to physician's offices in 2014 (the most recent year for which data are available; CDC 2016e).

Hippocrates is also credited with recognizing a second type of viral infection (again without realizing its cause or mode of transmission): hepatitis. The symptoms described by Hippocrates—"jaundice, dropsy, pale and foul-smelling stools, fever, itching, rumbling of the intestine and upper abdominal pain"—would be familiar to a clinician today for one form of the disease. Although Hippocrates himself called the infection thus described *epidemic jaundice*, its modern name actually comes from his basic description of the disease, "infection of the liver," from *hepatos* ("of the liver") and *itis* ("infection"; Mammas and Spandidos 2016). Today, six forms of hepatitis are recognized, one of which (hepatitis B) is the sixth most common STI in the United States (Tidy 2014).

The first virus to be isolated and definitively associated with disease was the tobacco mosaic virus, found in 1892 by Russian botanist Dmitri Ivanovski (also Ivanovsky). As its name suggests, it is the causative agent for a disease that affects tobacco plants and other members of the Solanaceae family. In short order, a number of other viruses were also found, including those responsible for foot-and-mouth disease (Loeffler and Frosch, 1898), African horse sickness (M'adyean, 1900), yellow fever (Reed et al., 1900–1901), rabies (Remlinger, 1903), canine distemper (Carré, Laidlaw, and Dunkin, 1905), poliomyelitis (Landsteiner and Popper, 1909), measles (Goldberger, et al., 1911), rubella (Hess, 1914; Hiro and Tasaka, 1938), and the first encephalitis virus (Breinl, Cleland, and French, 1918) (Oldstone 1998, Table 2.1, 21–22).

Herpes

The first virus associated with an STI was discovered in 1919 by German pathologist A. Löwenstein. Löwenstein removed the fluid from herpes infections of the eyes and lips from human patients and transferred it to the eyes of experimental rabbits. When the rabbits also developed herpes-like symptoms, Löwenstein concluded that a substance present in the original fluid was responsible for the disease, a substance later identified as the herpes simplex virus (HSV). Löwenstein's experiments were actually very similar to those of his colleague, W. Grüter, who had conducted a similar line of research nearly a decade earlier, but had failed to publish his results. Löwenstein acknowledged Grüter's contributions to his own work (da Fano 1923; Sawtell and Thompson 2016; Löwenstein's original article was Löwenstein 1919).

By the late 1950s, researchers had begun to discover that two types of HSVs exist, eventually designated as HSV-1 and HSV-2 (Figueroa and Rawls 1969, 259). At first—and for many years thereafter—they thought that two different viruses caused the two primary forms of herpes: the very common "cold sores" that occur primarily on the mouth and lips (HSV-1) and the form that causes lesions and other sores in the genital region (HSV-2). This line of thought led to somewhat different interpretations of the two infections. HSV-1 was thought to be responsible for rather mild, inconvenient, and unpleasant—but generally harmless and short-lived—infections. By contrast, HSV-2 was believed to cause an infection that was very painful and long-lasting in a region about which people did not like to talk, the genitals.

Today we know that this differentiation is far too simplistic. While cold sores *are* most commonly caused by HSV-1 and genital herpes by HSV-2, either virus may occur in either location. One very significant consequence of that finding is that herpes is rather easily transmitted between two individuals during oral sex, when a viral infection on the mouth becomes responsible for a similar infection (with the same virus) in the genital region. Another matter of concern is the tendency to take an HSV-1 (cold sore) too lightly, as a nuisance rather than a serious medical problem. But, in fact, one of the potential consequences of an HSV-1, "cold sore" infection is the possibility of the virus' migrating to the eyes, where it may cause ocular herpes, which, in turn, is a cause of blindness (STD Project 2017).

Hepatitis

The first form of hepatitis to be discovered and identified was the one currently known as hepatitis B. The story behind this discovery is of considerable interest and illustrates the role of chance in scientific research. In the late 1950s, American medical researcher Baruch Blumberg became interested in the possibility that a person's genetic background may be a factor in his or her tendency to contract various infectious diseases. In support of his research, he collected blood samples from a vast variety of individuals from all parts of the world. As his research developed, it became clear that some disease patterns could not adequately be explained by differences in genetic makeup among individuals. They could, however, be the result of previous exposure to various types of diseases. Sidetracked into this line of research, Blumberg and his colleagues eventually discovered the causative agent of the disease to be a new type of virus, now known as the hepatitis B virus (HBV). (Hepatitis B was originally known as *serum hepatitis* because of its association with blood.) Only two years later, Blumberg and a colleague, Irving Milliman, also invented the first vaccine against a viral disease, one designed to prevent hepatitis B. For his research on the virus, Blumberg received a share of the 1976 Nobel Prize in medicine or physiology (Patlak 2000).

Long before the discovery of HBV, medical workers were well aware of another form of hepatitis, one that seemed to be easily transmitted among groups of individuals living or working in close contact with each other, such as military groups. At first the disease was called *catarrhal, epidemic, or sporadic jaundice,* but by World War II, was more commonly known as *infectious hepatitis.* The causative agent for this form of hepatitis was discovered in 1973 by American virologists Stephen Feinstone, Albert Kapikian, and Robert H. Purcell (Feinstone, Kapikian, and Purcell 1973). The researchers discovered a new type of viral particle in the feces of individuals infected with infectious hepatitis and proved that it was the organism by which the disease was transmitted among people. That virus particle is now known as the hepatitis A virus (HAV; Cuthbert 2001).

Four other forms of hepatitis are also now known. The naming system adopted for the viruses involved has nothing to do with the chronological order in which they were discovered. For example, as noted above, HBV was discovered before HAV. The additional hepatitis viruses are summarized in Table 1.3.

Table 1.3 Summary of Hepatitis Viruses

Name	Discovery	Characteristics
HAV	Feinstone, Kapikian, and Purcell, 1973	Highly contagious; spread by fecal to oral contact, most commonly in crowded conditions with poor sanitation. Generally no liver damage and no repeated outbreaks. Vaccine available. 2,500 cases in the United States in 2014.
HBV	Blumberg, 1965	Spread through bodily fluids, such as blood and semen, through sexual contact, sharing of needles, during birth, and other means. May be mild and brief or long-lasting and life-threatening. Vaccine available. 19,200 cases in the United States in 2014.
HCV	Houghton, Choo, Kuo, and Bradley, 1989	Spread primarily through blood. Most common means of transmission today is sharing of needles or other drug paraphernalia. Risk of transmission by sexual contact is low. May be mild and brief or long-lasting and life-threatening. No vaccine available. 30,500 cases in the United States in 2014.
HDV	Rizzetto, 1977	Transmission primarily through sexual contact, needle sticks, and birth canal exposure. Occurs most commonly in connection with HBV. If untreated may lead to cirrhosis of the liver with serious consequences. Rare in the United States.

(continued)

Table 1.3   (Continued)

Name	Discovery	Characteristics
HEV	Balayan, Andjaparidze, Savinskaya, Ketiladze, Braginsky, Savinov, and Poleschuk, 1983	Rare in the United States, but common in developing countries worldwide. Transmitted by fecal-oral contact or through contaminated food. Most commonly brief and mild, but may lead to chronic, more serious forms of hepatitis.
HFV	none	An hypothesized form for which no experimental evidence is yet available.
HGV	Simons et al., 1995; Linnen et al., 1996	Fairly common in the United States and worldwide, with prevalence rates of about 3%. Little or no evidence of a connection between HGV and any form of hepatitis.

Human Papillomavirus

The most common STI in the United States today is HPV. Reliable data about the prevalence and incidence of the disease are difficult to obtain since it is not a legally reportable condition in the United States. According to one recent estimate, however, about 79 million Americans are currently infected with the virus, and 14 million more are being infected annually (CDC 2017; Hariri et al. 2014). The disease can be transmitted through oral, anal, or genital sex with someone who has the virus. The vast majority of infections are asymptomatic, so that infected individuals usually are not even aware that they have the disease. In about 90 percent of all cases, the infection disappears within a period of about two years without any serious health effects to an individual. The most important exception to that pattern, however, results from the fact that HPV is strongly implicated in the development of cervical cancer. About 70 percent of all cervical cancers worldwide are thought to have been caused by one or another form of the HPV (Hariri et al. 2014).

Progress toward the discovery of HPV and its association with cervical cancer has a long and fascinating history. One of the earliest episodes in that story took place in 1842 when the Italian physician Domenico Antonio Rigoni-Stern hypothesized that some forms of cancer might be caused by an infectious agent. Rigoni-Stern based his hypothesis on the fact that his own research showed that married women whom he had treated were far more likely to develop cervical cancer than were nuns (although nuns were much more likely to die of breast cancer). Rigoni-Stern suggested that this difference could be explained by the fact that married women were sexually active, and could, therefore, pick up an infectious agent than were nuns (Rigoni-Stern 1987).

The search for a transmissible agent responsible for cervical cancer went on for well over a century, with a number of relatively modest, but essential, breakthroughs registered from time to time. A key step in this process occurred in the early 1930s when American researcher Richard E. Shope discovered a particle that met Rigoni-Stern's hypothesis, a virus now called the cottontail rabbit papillomavirus (CRPV). That discovery came about when Shope heard about a particularly unusual type of rabbit found in the American West called *jackalopes*. The name came from the fact that these rabbits had large warts on their head that looked like horns. Shope was able to extract material from these ground-up warts that he then transferred to normal, non-horned rabbits. As a result of that procedure the normal rabbits themselves also began to develop tumors ("horns") (Kaylin 2006).

Shope's research was of great significance, not only to researchers who study rabbits, but also to those who were looking for a connection between transmissible materials and human cancer. Almost certainly, the most important of the researchers inspired by Shope's work was German virologist Harald zur Hausen. Zur Hausen had been interested in the relationship between infectious diseases and cancer since the earliest years of his academic career. Lacking the formal background to conduct the needed studies, however, he struggled for a number of years obtaining the basic information he needed to conduct this research and finding a setting in which he could work on precisely the problem in which he was interested.

One of his first discoveries is that HPV occurs in common plantar warts experienced by many people, thus confirming that Shope's results also applied to humans. The next important breakthrough provided the key he needed to make his final discovery: that HPV actually occurs in a number of different subtypes (about 40 of which are now known) that have differing effects on the human body. In fact, the discovery of subtype HPV-16 in 1983 and HPV-18 a year later provided the missing piece of the puzzle. Efforts to detect the more common forms of HPV, such as HPV-6, in cervical cancers had proved to be unsuccessful. But when zur Hausen turned his attention to the newly discovered HPV-16 and HPV-18, he had much greater success: both subtypes were present in the cancers, suggesting that they, indeed, were the causative agent for the disease. Zur Hausen was later awarded a share of the 2008 Nobel Prize in medicine or physiology for his work on HPV and cervical cancer (Norkin 2015; Zur Hausen 2009).

Human Immunodeficiency Virus

A second viral STI of major significance has been HIV/AIDS. The term *HIV/AIDS* stands for *human immunodeficiency virus*, the causative agent of the disease, and *acquired immune deficiency syndrome*, the name of the disease itself. HIV/AIDS was first reported in the United States in the early 1980s, and eventually spread widely throughout the gay and drug-using community. According to the most recent data available, 1,194,039 people in the United States were diagnosed with AIDS between 1981 and 2013, of whom 658,507 died. As of early 2016, more than 1.2 million people in the United States were infected with HIV, about 12 percent of whom are thought not to be aware of their HIV status. Worldwide, an estimated 78 million people contracted AIDS since the early 1980s, of whom about 35 million have died. An estimated 36.7 million people were living with HIV in 2016, the majority of whom were in sub-Saharan Africa. An estimated 2.1 million people were becoming infected annually in 2015 (Statistic: Worldwide 2017).

Progress in dealing with HIV/AIDS was slow at first, at least partly because the individuals most at risk for the infection—gay men and drug users—were held in low esteem by most Americans. In fact, early on in the epidemic, President Ronald Reagan's press secretary Larry Speakes spoke laughingly of the condition at a press conference, suggesting that a questioner from the press might be gay himself for even knowing about the disease (Stern 2015; contains audio of press conference involved). Reagan himself never mentioned the disease in a forum public until May 31, 1987, at which point more than 25,000 Americans had already died of the disease (Specter 2016). One consequence of this inattention to the disease was that funding for research was difficult to obtain, and progress in understanding HIV/AIDS occurred only very slowly. (Among the many books and articles on this point, see especially Shilts 1987.)

The two primary research centers on the causative agent of HIV were the Pasteur Institute in Paris, under the direction of French virologist Luc Montagnier, and Laboratory for Tumor Cell Biology at the National Cancer Institute, under the direction of virologist Robert Gallo. In 1983, Montagnier announced the discovery of a virus associated with the occurrence of HIV that he called the *lymphadenopathy-associated virus* (LAV). A year later, Gallo also reported finding a virus that he believed was the cause of HIV, a virus he named the *human T-lymphotropic virus*, or HTLV-III. For some time, the two laboratories argued as to which should receive credit for making the discovery of the new virus, that was eventually renamed the human immunodeficiency virus (HIV), a dispute that has become famous as one of the most contentious debates in modern medical science. Eventually that debate was resolved in June 1984 when Montagnier and Gallo appeared at a joint press conference in which they reported that LAV and HTLV-III were almost certainly the same organism. Almost a decade later, they confirmed this position in a joint paper published in *The New England Journal of Medicine* in 2003 (Gallo and

Montagnier 2003; for a summary of the research on HIV, see Office of NIH History 2017). The dispute between Gallo and Montagnier was revisited in 2008 when Montagnier—but not Gallo—was awarded a share of the Nobel Prize in physiology or medicine for his discovery of HIV.

Today, no cure for HIV has yet been discovered, nor are vaccines available to prevent occurrence of the disease. However, some effective treatment regimens have been developed allowing infected individuals to live relatively normal lives. As noted at the beginning of this section, however, the disease is still rampant in many parts of the world and is widely regarded as one of the planet's most serious public health problems.

Diagnosis and Treatment

The discovery of the causative agent of various STIs was, of course, more than an impressive research achievement. This new information also opened up whole new areas of the diagnosis, prevention, and treatment of the infections involved. For example, the discovery of *T. pallidum* in 1905 was followed almost immediately by the development of a variety of methods by which syphilis could be diagnosed. It was no longer necessary for a health care worker to guess about the cause of a person's signs and symptoms; specific tests had become available allowing a positive identification of the disease. (For a review of some of these early tests, see Bialynicki-Birula 2008; CDC 1998; The Great Pox 2007.) Perhaps the most famous of these early diagnostic techniques was the so-called Wassermann test, named after one of its discoverers, German bacteriologist August Paul von Wassermann, who worked with Albert Neisser on the test.

At one time, the Wassermann test was widely used for the diagnosis of syphilis. Perhaps its most common application was as a requirement for the issuance of a marriage certificate. For much of the 20th century, every state in the United States required such a test to obtain a marriage license. Today, such tests no longer exist in any state in the Union or the District of Columbia (Chart: State Marriage License and Blood Test Requirements 2017).

The discovery of the causative agent for STIs also provided a strong impetus for the development of new methods for treating those diseases. Among the leading researchers in this field was German biochemist Paul Ehrlich. As early as 1891, Ehrlich had suggested a new method for treating infectious diseases to replace the traditional trial-and-error approach of simple testing one treatment after another. Ehrlich suggested that once the causative agent of an infectious disease had been identified, it should be possible to find a specific chemical compound, a "magic bullet," that was capable of attacking and destroying that agent. Ehrlich's concept formed the basis of modern chemotherapy, the use of chemical substances to treat disease. His earliest research involved the use of the dye methylene blue to treat malaria, a line of research that was only moderately successful.

He then proceeded to explore the use of a variety of compounds of arsenic to treat trypanosomal infections (diseases caused by bacteria of the genus *Trypanosoma*). He achieved some success in this pursuit, although the toxicity of arsenic sometimes caused more damage than good. It was while he was working on this line of research that Ehrlich heard about the discovery of *T. pallidum* and switched his attention to a search for a chemical—a "magic bullet"—that would destroy the *T. pallidum* bacterium.

In 1909, Ehrlich, along with his colleague Japanese bacteriologist Sahachiro Hata, announced the discovery of the first effective chemotherapeutic agent for the treatment of syphilis, an arsenic-containing compound originally called simply *606* (because it was the 606th compound they tested), but later given the name of *salvarsan*. In a process that would startle modern-day pharmaceutical researches, salvarsan was made available for commercial use within less than a year and quickly became the drug of choice for treating syphilis (Bosch and Rosicha 2008).

The discovery of salvarsan and its somewhat improved analog, neosalvaran, developed by Ehrlich in 1914, marked a turning point in the treatment of STIs. For the first time, a dependable, safe, effective method for curing an STI was available to the medical community. And for more than three decades, these compounds remained the treatment of choice for syphilis. In 1928, however, another alternative became available: penicillin.

The story of the accidental discovery of the first antibiotic by British bacteriologist Sir Alexander Fleming is now probably too well known to be repeated here (Markel 2013). The irony of that great event was that Fleming himself was ill-equipped to advance the development of penicillin for the treatment of infections, having neither the background in chemistry nor the financial resources to continue his research with the drug. In fact, it was not until a decade later that another British researcher, pathologist Howard Florey, began studies of the effects of penicillin on infections in mice and discovered that the substance was remarkably effective in preventing and curing otherwise deadly streptococcal infections.

It quickly became obvious that the drug might also be effective in the treatment of a variety of other infections in humans as well as in laboratory animals. And on February 12, 1941, a 43-year-old British policeman named Albert Alexander became the first human to be treated with penicillin. A scratch incurred while trimming his roses soon became infected, and Alexander rapidly became very ill. None of the available anti-infectives was effective in treating the problem, and his doctors decided to try penicillin. The treatment worked, and the place of the new drug in the arsenal of modern medicine had been established.

The use of penicillin against syphilis did not become popular, however, until World War II when the U.S. military establishment desperately began a search for a quick, inexpensive, and effective treatment for syphilis among draftees and active members of the armed services. A series of experiments conducted in 1943 by physicians John F. Mahoney, R. C. Arnold, and Ad Harris found that the use of penicillin provided the cure for which the armed services had been looking. At last, a treatment that was both safe and effective against perhaps the most serious of all STIs to that date in human history had been found (Frith 2012; Mahoney, Arnold, and Harris 1943).

Penicillin's success against syphilis soon led to its use against other bacterial forms of STIs, such as gonorrhea and chlamydia. By the 1970s, however, clinicians began to see a troubling change in the effectiveness of penicillin against these and other infections. The causative agents responsible for the infections had begun to mutate into forms that were more resistant to penicillin, gradually reaching a point where even larger and larger doses of the drug were ineffective in curing the disease. At that point, a cat-and-mouse game began that is now familiar to medical researchers: new drugs, chemically close relatives of penicillin, were devised that were more effective than penicillin itself, thereby providing a new treatment to replace the older one. Before long, microorganisms continued to mutate, developing immunity this time against the "new and better" penicillin substitutes. This situation led to the development of other families of drugs capable of destroying the bacteria that cause STIs. Those bacteria that also eventually became resistant to the new families of antibiotics required even further research on new treatments for STIs. Thus, over time, medical workers have had to continue adjusting their treatments, turning to drugs such as azithromycin, doxycycline, erythromycin, metronidazole, ofloxacin, and tetracycline for the treatment of STIs.

The great fear among STI researchers has always been that causative agents will eventually win this battle, and that researchers will be unable to find new products to combat their actions. Such has become very nearly the case today with regard to gonorrheal infections. In 2013, the CDC announced that the *N. gonorrhoeae* bacterium had become resistant to all traditional forms of treatments—sulfonilamides, penicillin, tetracycline, and fluoroquinolones—and that only one class of antibiotics, the cephalosporins, was still effective in the treatment of gonorrhea. The CDC noted in its announcement that "given the bacteria's ability to adapt and survive antibiotics, it is critical to continuously monitor for antibiotic resistance and encourage research and development of new treatment regimens for gonorrhea" (CDC 2016a).

Vaccines

One of the questions one might ask about STIs is why there are not more vaccines for these infections. After all, researchers have developed vaccines for nearly 30 other infectious diseases, including measles, mumps, tetanus, rubella, cholera, anthrax, tuberculosis, poliomyelitis, yellow fever, and rabies. But as of late 2017, vaccines are available for only three STIs: hepatitis A, hepatitis B, and the HPV. The first of these vaccines, for hepatitis B, was developed in 1969 by American geneticist Baruch Blumberg and his coworkers, while the hepatitis A vaccine became commercially available in the United States in 1995 and the HPV vaccine in 2006 (Patlak 2000; Martine and Lemon 2006; Smith 2014).

One reason that more vaccines are not available for STIs is that simple, inexpensive, and effective treatments for many of them are currently available. So the enormous cost of developing a vaccine is not really justified. Another reason is that the technical problems involved in developing a vaccine are so great that success has thus far been elusive. For example, researchers have for at least two decades been searching for a vaccine against HIV that would dramatically reduce the incidence of that disease. But the virus appears to be so "clever" (i.e., it evolves so rapidly) that no vaccine has yet been found to stay ahead of the rate at which it changes properties. Still, the search for vaccines for HIV, chlamydia, genital herpes, and other STIs continues, with varying degrees of progress and possible success (Anna 2015).

Conclusion

To an observer at the turn of the 21st century, the outlook for prevention and treatment of STIs would appear to be very bright. Researchers had learned—and were continuing to discover—many of the most basic facts about these infections, the organisms that cause them, and the ways in which they can be diagnosed, prevented, and treated. The preceding century had appeared to be a story of one conquest over STIs after another.

But the second decade of the new century offered a quite different view. In its Sexually Transmitted Disease Surveillance Report for 2015, released in October 2016, the CDC summarized data showing that such diseases had reached "an unprecedented high" in the United States. In commenting on the report, Dr. Jonathan Mermin, director of the CDC National Center for HIV/AIDS, Viral Hepatitis, STD, and TB Prevention, said that the country "had reached a decisive moment" in which the "country's systems for preventing STDs had eroded," creating the potential that the nation's "human and economic burden will continue to grow" (CDC 2016c). The changes that have occurred in the status of STIs in the United States, the factors that have led to those changes, and the steps that can and must be taken to reverse this course are the topic of Chapter 2 of this book.

References

Albritton, W. L. 1989. "Biology of *Haemophilus ducreyi*." *Microbiological Reviews,* 53(4): 377–389.

American Sexual Health Association. 2016. "STDs/STIs." http://www.ashasexualhealth.org/stdsstis/. Accessed on February 2, 2017.

Anna C. 2015. "STD Awareness: Which STDs Are Vaccine Preventable?" Planned Parenthood. http://advocatesaz.org/2015/08/17/

std-awareness-which-stds-are-vaccine-preventable/. Accessed on February 2, 2017.

Arrizabalaga, Jon, John Henderson, and Roger French. 1997. *The Great Pox: The French Disease in Renaissance Europe*. New Haven, CT: Yale University Press.

Asimov, Isaac. 1982. *Asimov's Biographical Encyclopedia of Science and Technology*, 2nd rev. ed. Garden City, NY: Doubleday. http://emilkirkegaard.dk/en/wp-content/uploads/Asimovs%20Biographical%20Encyclopedia%20of%20Science%20and%20Technology%20Isaac%20Asimov%20941p.pdf. Accessed on February 24, 2017.

Ayoade, Folusakin O. 2017. "Herpes Simplex." Medscape. https://emedicine.medscape.com/article/218580-overview. Accessed on November 7, 2017.

Bardell, David. 2004. "The Invention of the Microscope." *Bios,* 75(2): 78–84.

Barnett, James A. 2008. "A History of Research on Yeasts 12: Medical Yeasts, Part I, *Candida albicans.*" *Yeast,* 25(6): 385–417.

Benedek, Thomas G. n.d. "Albert L. Neisser (1855–1916), Microbiologist and Venereologist." antimicrobe.org. Available at http://www.antimicrobe.org/h04c.files/history/Neisser.pdf. Accessed on February 17, 2017.

Benedek, Thomas G. 2014. "'Case Neisser': Experimental Design, the Beginnings of Immunology, and Informed Consent." *Perspectives in Biology and Medicine,* 57(2): 249–267.

Bialynicki-Birula, Rafal. 2008. "The 100th Anniversary of Wassermann–Neisser–Bruck Reaction." *Clinics in Dermatology,* 26(1): 79–88.

Black, Carolyn M. 2013. "Introduction." In Carolyn M. Black, ed. *Chlamydial Infection: A Clinical and Public Health Perspective*. Basel: Karger.

Bosch, Fèlix, and Laia Rosicha. 2008. "The Contributions of Paul Ehrlich to Pharmacology: A Tribute on the Occasion of the Centenary of His Nobel Prize." *Pharmacology,* 82(3): 171–179.

Boskey, Elizabeth. 2016. "The Incubation Period of Common STDs." verywell. Available at https://www.verywell.com/how-long-before-std-symptoms-appear-3133026. Accessed on March 7, 2017.

Bradley, Richard. 1721. *The Plague at Marseilles Consider'd: With Remarks upon the Plague in General, Shewing Its Cause and Nature of Infection, with Necessary Precautions to Prevent the Spreading of That Direful Distemper.* Dublin: J. Carson. https://books.google.com/books?id=FtpbAAAAQAAJ&q=poisonous+insects#v=onepage&q=microscope&f=false. Accessed on February 25, 2017.

Brittain, C. Dale. 2015. "Life in the Middle Ages: Medieval Brothels." http://cdalebrittain.blogspot.com/2015/02/medieval-brothels.html. Accessed on February 4, 2017.

Burg, G. 2012. "History of Sexually Transmitted Infections (STI)." *Giornale Italiano di Dermatologia e Venereologia,* 147(4): 329–340.

Celsus. 1935. *De Medicina.* Trans. by Walter George Spencer. The Perseus Catalog, Book 6, Chapter 18. http://www.perseus.tufts.edu/hopper/text?doc=Perseus:abo:phi,0836,002:6:18. Accessed on February 4, 2017.

Centers for Disease Control and Prevention. 1998. "History of Diagnostic Tests for Syphilis." https://www.cdc.gov/std/syphilis/manual-1998/chapt1a2.pdf. Accessed on February 1, 2017.

Centers for Disease Control and Prevention. 2016a. "Antibiotic Resistant Gonorrhea Basic Information." https://www.cdc.gov/std/gonorrhea/arg/basic.htm. Accessed on February 1, 2017.

Centers for Disease Control and Prevention. 2016b. "Invasive Candidiasis Statistics." https://www.cdc.gov/fungal/ diseases/candidiasis/invasive/statistics.html. Accessed on February 17, 2017.

Centers for Disease Control and Prevention. 2016c. "Reported STDs at Unprecedented Highs in the U.S." 2016. https://www.cdc.gov/nchhstp/newsroom/2016/ std-surveillance-report-2015-press-release.html. Accessed on February 2, 2017.

Centers for Disease Control and Prevention. 2016d. "Table 1. Sexually Transmitted Diseases—Reported Cases and Rates of Reported Cases per 100,000 Population, United States, 1941–2015." 2016. https://www.cdc.gov/std/stats15/ tables/1.htm. Accessed on February 18, 2017.

Centers for Disease Control and Prevention. 2016e. "Table 44. Selected STDs and Complications—Initial Visits to Physicians' Offices, National Disease and Therapeutic Index, United States, 1966-2014." Available at https://www.cdc.gov/std/stats15/tables/44.htm. Accessed on February 19, 2017.

Centers for Disease Control and Prevention. 2016f. "2015 Sexually Transmitted Diseases Surveillance." 2016. https:// www.cdc.gov/std/stats15/tables/1.htm. Accessed on February 17, 2017.

Centers for Disease Control and Prevention. 2017. "Genital HPV Infection—Fact Sheet." https://www.cdc.gov/std/ hpv/stdfact-hpv.htm. Accessed on February 21, 2017.

Chandrasekar, Pranatharthi Haran. 2016. "Syphilis." Medscape. http://emedicine.medscape.com/article/229461 -overview#showall. Accessed on February 9, 2017.

"Chart: State Marriage License and Blood Test Requirements." 2017. Nolo. http://www.nolo.com/legal-encyclopedia/ chart-state-marriage-license-blood-29019.html. Accessed on February 1, 2017.

Choi, Charles Q. 2011. "Case Closed? Columbus Introduced Syphilis to Europe." LiveScience/Scientific American. https://www.scientificamerican.com/article/case-closed-columbus/. Accessed on February 9, 2017.

Cuthbert, Jennifer A. 2001. "Hepatitis A: Old and New." *Clinical Microbiology Reviews,* 14(1): 38–58. https://www.ncbi.nlm.nih.gov/pmc/articles/PMC88961/#B78. Accessed on February 20, 2017.

da Fano, Corrado Donato. 1923. "Herpetic Meningo-encephalitis in Rabbits." *The Journal of Pathology.* http://onlinelibrary.wiley.com/doi/10.1002/path.1700260112/abstract. Accessed on February 20, 2017.

Diamantis, Aristidis, Emmanouil Magiorkinis, and George Androutsos. 2009. "Alfred François Donné (1801–78): A Pioneer of Microscopy, Microbiology and Haematology." *Journal of Medical Biography,* 17(2): 81–87.

Donné A. F. 1836. "Animalcules Observés Dans La Matière Purulente et Leproduit Des Secretions Des Organs Génitaux De L'homme et De Lafemme." *Comptes Rendus Hebdomadaires des Séances de l'Academie des Sciences,* 3: 385–386 (in French).

Echeverria, Virginia Iommi. 2010. "Girolamo Fracastoro and the Invention of Syphilis." *Historia, Ciencias, Saude—Manguinhos,* 17(4): 877–884.

Fanoni, Antonio. 1905. "The Spirochæta Pallida in Syphilis." *New York Medical Journal and Philadelphia Medical Journal,* 82: 944. https://books.google.com/books?id=_olMAQAAMAAJ&pg=PA945&lpg=PA945&dq=syphilis+1905+hoffman+schaudinn&source=bl&ots=sHKq4nmK2X&sig=aOFu6ENjW9ngrOQ6_pDxq1fur2Y&hl=en&sa=X&ved=0ahUKEwiVpNKg0aHRAhWLy4MKHVXiABw4ChDoAQgfMAE#v=onepage&q=siegel&f=false.

Feinstone, Stephen M., Albert Z. Kapikian, and Robert H. Purcell. 1973. "Hepatitis A: Detection by Immune

Electron Microscopy of a Viruslike Antigen Associated with Acute Illness." *Science,* 182(4116): 1026–1028.

Figueroa, M. E., and W. E. Rawls. 1969. "Biological Markers for Differentiation of Herpes-virus Strains of Oral and Genital Origin." *Journal of General Virology,* 4: 259–267. http://www.microbiologyresearch.org/docserver/fulltext/jgv/4/2/JV0040020259.pdf?expires=1483658409&id=id&accname=guest&checksum=0DEF4F3151202E00C89AD D1FD187519A. Accessed on February 20, 2017.

Frith, John. 2012. "Syphilis—Its Early History and Treatment until Penicillin, and the Debate on Its Origins." *Journal of Military and Veterans Health,* 20(4): 49–58. http://jmvh.org/article/syphilis-its-early-history-and-treatment-until-penicillin-and-the-debate-on-its-origins/. Accessed on February 9, 2017.

Gallo, Robert C., and Luc Montagnier. 2003. "The Discovery of HIV as the Cause of AIDS." *The New England Journal of Medicine,* 349(24): 2283–2285.

"Gonorrhea—What Happens?" 2017. WebMD. http://www.webmd.com/sexual-conditions/tc/gonorrhea-what-happens. Accessed on February 12, 2017.

"The Great Pox." 2007. IBMS Congress. (Search for this item on your search engine for access to this article.)

Grimes, D. Jay. 2006. "Koch's Postulates—Then and Now." *Microbe,* 1(5): 223–228.

Gruber, Franjo, Jasna Lipozenčić, and Tatjana Kehler. 2015. "History of Venereal Diseases from Antiquity to the Renaissance." *Acta Dermatovenerologica Croatica,* 23(1): 1–11. hrcak.srce.hr/file/204588. Accessed on February 3, 2017.

Hariri, Susan, et al. 2014. "Human Papillomavirus (HPV)." Centers for Disease Control and Prevention. https://www.cdc.gov/vaccines/pubs/surv-manual/chpt05-hpv.html. Accessed on February 21, 2017.

Harper, Kristin N., et al. 2008. "On the Origin of the Treponematoses: A Phylogenetic Approach." *PLoS Neglected Tropical Diseases,* 2(1): e148. http://journals.plos. org/plosntds/article?id=10.1371/journal.pntd.0000148#pn td-0000148-t002. Accessed on February 9, 2017.

"Healing Prayer for Sexually Transmitted Diseases, Herpes, Syphilis and AIDS John Mellor Healing." 2015. YouTube. https://www.youtube.com/watch?v=HgfGrsCLNfQ. Accessed on February 11, 2017

Hippocrates. 2009. "Of the Epidemics." Trans. by Francis Adams. *The Internet Classics Archive.* http://classics.mit.edu/ Hippocrates/epidemics.1.i.html. Accessed on February 4, 2017.

International Trachoma Initiative. 2015. "The World's Leading Cause of Preventable Blindness." http://trachoma. org/about-trachoma. Accessed on February 18, 2017.

Karamanou, Marianna, et al. 2012. "From Miasmas to Germs: A Historical Approach to Theories of Infectious Disease Transmission." *Le Infezioni in Medicina: Rivista Periodica Di Eziologia, Epidemiologia, Diagnostica, Clinica E Terapia Delle Patologie Infettive,* 20(1): 58–62. https://www.researchgate. net/publication/223957556_From_miasmas_to_germs_A_ historical_approach_to_theories_of_infectious_disease_ transmission. Accessed on February 11, 2017.

Kaylin, Jennifer. 2006. "The Virus behind the Cancer." *Yale Medicine,* 40(2). http://yalemedicine.yale.edu/spring2006/ features/feature/52007/. Accessed on February 21, 2017.

LaCroix, Paul, and Samuel Putnam. 1931. *History of Prostitution.* Vol. 2. Whitefish, MT: Kessinger Publishing. https://archive.org/details/LacroixPHistoryOfProstitution AmongAllThePeoplesOfTheWorldFromTheMostRemote Antiqu_201707. Accessed on November 7, 2017.

Lende, Daniel. 2010. "Gonorrhea and the Clap: The Slap Down Treatment." PLOS Blogs. http://

blogs.plos.org/neuroanthropology/2010/09/17/
gonorrhea-and-the-clap-the-slap-down-treatment/.
Accessed on February 10, 2017.

Löwenstein, A. 1919. "Aetiologische Untersuchungen uber
den Fieberhaften, Herpes." ["Etiological Studies on
Febrile, Herpes."] *Munchener Medizinische Wochenschrift*,
66:769–770.

Macedo de Souza, Elemir. 2005. "Há 100 Anos, a Descoberta
do Treponema pallidum." *Anais Brasileiros de Dermatologia*,
80(5): 547–548. http://www.scielo.br/pdf/abd/v80n5/
en_v80n5a17.pdf (in English). Accessed on February 17,
2017.

Mahoney, John F., R. C. Arnold, and Ad Harris. 1943.
"Penicillin Treatment of Early Syphilis: A Preliminary
Report." *American Journal of Public Health and the Nation's
Health*, 33(12): 1387–1391.

Mammas, Ioannis N., and Deterios A. Spandidos. 2016.
"Paediatric Virology in the Hippocratic Corpus."
Experimental and Therapeutic Medicine, 12(2): 541–
549. https://www.ncbi.nlm.nih.gov/pmc/articles/
PMC4950906/. Accessed on February 19, 2017.

Mardh, Otilla, Ninnie Abrahamsson, and Andrew Amato-
Gauci. 2016. "Chancroid—A Rare Disease in Europe?"
in Slide Share. http://www.slideshare.net/ECDC_EU/
chancroid-a-reare-disease-in-europe-iusti-europe-i2016.
Accessed on February 21, 2017.

Markel, Howard. 2013. "The Real Story behind Penicillin."
PBS Newshour. http://www.pbs.org/newshour/rundown/
the-real-story-behind-the-worlds-first-antibiotic/. Accessed
on February 22, 2017.

Martine, Annette, and Stanley M. Lemon. 2006. "Hepatitis
A Virus: From Discovery to Vaccines." *Hepatology*, 43(S1):
S164-S172. http://onlinelibrary.wiley.com/doi/10.1002/
hep.21052/full. Accessed on February 2, 2017.

McDonnell, Robert, ed. 1881. *Selections from the Works of Abraham Colles, Consisting Chiefly of His Practical Observations on the Venereal Disease, and on the Use of Mercury.* London: The New Sydenham Society. https:// archive.org/stream/selectionsfromwo00colluoft/ selectionsfromwo00colluoft_djvu.txt. Accessed on February 11, 2017.

Moore, Wendy. 2009. "John Hunter (1728–1793)." The James Lind Library. http://www.jameslindlibrary.org/ articles/john-hunter-1728-93/. Accessed on February 11, 2017.

Morton, R. S. 1991. "Sexual Attitudes, Preferences and Infections in Ancient Greece: Has Antiquity Anything Useful for Us Today?" *Genitourinary Medicine,* 67(1): 59–66. https://www.ncbi.nlm.nih.gov/pmc/articles/ PMC1194618/pdf/genitmed00037-0065.pdf. Accessed on November 7, 2017.

Noguchi, Hideyo, and J. W. Moore. 1913. "A Demonstration of Treponema Pallidum in the Brain in Cases of General Paralysis." *Journal of Experimental Medicine,* 17(2): 232–238. http://jem.rupress.org/content/jem/17/2/232.full.pdf. Accessed on February 17, 2017.

Norkin, Leonard. 2015. "Harald zur Hausen, Papillomaviruses, and Cervical Cancer." https:// norkinvirology.wordpress.com/2015/06/19/ harold-zur-hausen-papillomaviruses-and-cervical-cancer/. Accessed on November 7, 2017.

Norris, Charles Cambios. 1913. *Gonorrhea in Women: Its Pathology, Symptomatology, Diagnosis, and Treatment; Together with a Review of the Rare Varieties of the Disease Which Occur in Men, Women and Children.* Philadelphia; London: W. B. Saunders.

Nutton, Vivian. 1983. "The Seeds of Disease: An Explanation of Contagion and Infection from the Greeks to the

Renaissance." *Medical History,* 27(1): 1–34. https://
www.ncbi.nlm.nih.gov/pmc/articles/PMC1139262/pdf/
medhist00084-0005.pdf. Accessed on February 11, 2017.

Nutton, Vivian. 1990. "The Reception of Fracastoro's Theory
of Contagion: The Seed That Fell among Thorns?" *Osiris,*
6(1): 196–234.

Obladen, Michael. 2012. "Thrush—Nightmare of the
Foundling Hospitals." *Neonatology,* 101(3): 159–165.

Office of NIH History. 2017. "In Their Own Words: NIH
Researchers Recall the Early Years of AIDS." https://history.
nih.gov/nihinownwords/docs/page_29.html. Accessed on
February 2, 2017.

Oldstone, Michael B. A. 1998. *Viruses, Plagues, and History.*
New York: Oxford University Press.

Oriel, J. D. 1994. *The Scars of Venus: A History of Venereology.*
New York: Springer-Verlag.

Osborne, David K. 2015. Greek Medicine.net. http://www.
greekmedicine.net/whos_who/Galen.html. Accessed on
February 5, 2017.

Pàlfi, György, et al. 1992. "Pre-Columbian Congenital
Syphilis from the Late Antiquity in France." *International
Journal of Osteoarchaeology,* 2(3): 245–263.

Pashkov, Konstantin A., and Mikhail S. Betekhtin. 2014.
"Philippe Ricord—Prominent Venereologist of the
XIX Century." *History of Medicine,* 1(4): 9–12. http://
en.historymedjournal.com/volume/number_4/Histori_
medical_4-2014_english_Pashkov.pdf. Accessed on
February 11, 2017.

Patlak, Margie. 2000. "The Hepatiatis B Story." Beyond
Discovery. http://www.nasonline.org/publications/
beyond-discovery/hepatitis-b-story.pdf. Accessed on
February 20, 2017.

Paulissian, Robert. 1991. "Medicine in Ancient Assyria and
Babylonia." *Journal of Assyrian Academic Studies,* 5(1):

3–51. http://www.jaas.org/edocs/v5n1/Paulissian.pdf. Accessed on February 2, 2017.

Plumb, Brian. 1997. "Sexually Transmitted Diseases: An Historical Retrospect." http://www.evolve360.co.uk/ data/10/docs/10/10plumb.pdf. Accessed on February 3, 2017.

"Prayer for Healing of any Diseases and Sickness." 2017. Prayers for Special Help. http://www.prayers-for-special-help.com/ prayer-for-healing-of-any-diseases-and-sickness.html. Accessed on February 11, 2017.

Rao, T. V. 2017. "Spirochetes." Slide Player. http://slideplayer. com/slide/4642226/. Accessed on February 17, 2017.

Ricord, Ph. 1842. *A Practical Treatise on Venereal Diseases*. New York: P. Gordon. https://archive.org/ stream/100960314.nlm.nih.gov/100960314_djvu.txt. Accessed on February 11, 2017.

Rigoni-Stern. 1987. "Statistical Facts about Cancers on Which Doctor Rigoni-Stern Based His Contribution to the Surgeons' Subgroup of the IV Congress of the Italian Scientists on 23 September 1842." Trans. by Biancaw De Stavola. *Statistics in Medicine,* 6(8): 881–884.

Roizman, B., and R. J. Whitley. 2001. "The Nine Ages of Herpes Simplex Virus." *Herpes,* 8(1): 23–27.

Rosebury, Theodor. 1971. *Microbes and Morals; the Strange Story of Venereal Disease*. New York: Viking Press.

Rosenbaum, Julius. 1901. *The Plague of Lust, Being a History of Venereal Disease in Classical Antiquity,* 2 vols. Paris: Charles Carrington. https://archive.org/ details/plagueoflustbein01rose and https://archive.org/ details/plagueoflustbein02rose. Accessed on February 10, 2017.

Rothschild, Bruce M. 2005. "History of Syphilis." *Clinical Infectious Diseases,* 40(10): 1454–1463.

Sanger, Melvin. 2007. "How It Happened That a Portion of a Treatise Entitled 'New Improvements of Planting and Gardening Both Philosophical and Practical' by Richard Bradley FRS, Which Dealt with Blights of Trees and Plants, Provided the First Report of an Environment That Contained Green Sulphur Photosynthetic Bacteria." *Notes and Records of the Royal Society of London,* 61(3): 327–332. http://rsnr.royalsocietypublishing.org/content/61/3/327. Accessed on February 25, 2017.

Sawtell, Nancy M., and Richard L. Thompson. 2016. "Herpes Simplex Virus and the Lexicon of Latency and Reactivation: A Call for Defining Terms and Building an Integrated Collective Framework." F1000Res. doi: 10.12688/f1000research.8886.1. https://www.ncbi. nlm.nih.gov/pmc/articles/PMC4995687/. Accessed on February 20, 2017.

Schlagel, Richard H. 2010. *Seeking the Truth : How Science Has Prevailed over the Supernatural Worldview.* Amherst, NY: Humanity Books.

Scurlock, Jo Ann. 2014. *Sourcebook for Ancient Mesopotamian Medicine.* Atlanta: Society of Biblical Literature.

Scurlock, Jo Ann, and Burton R. Andersen. 2005. *Diagnoses in Assyrian and Babylonian Medicine: Ancient Sources, Translations, and Modern Medical Analyses.* Urbana: University of Illinois Press.

"Sexually Transmitted Diseases Treatment Guidelines, 2015." 2015. *Morbidity and Mortality Weekly Report,* 64(3). https://www.cdc.gov/Mmwr/pdf/rr/rr6403.pdf. Accessed on February 18, 2017.

Shilts, Randy. 1987. *And the Band Played On: Politics, People, and the AIDS Epidemic.* New York: St. Martin's Press.

Shim, Bong Suk. 2011. "Current Concepts in Bacterial Sexually Transmitted Diseases." *Korean Journal of Urology,* 52(9): 589–597. https://www.ncbi.nlm.

nih.gov/pmc/articles/PMC3198230/. Accessed on February 3, 2017.

Smith, Emma. 2014. "HPV: The Whole Story: Warts and All." Cancer Research UK. http://scienceblog. cancerresearchuk.org/2014/09/16/hpv-the-whole-story-war ts-and-all/. Accessed on February 2, 2017.

Specter, Michael. 2016. "Hillary Clinton, Nancy Reagan, and AIDS." *The New Yorker*. http://www.newyorker.com/news/ daily-comment/hillary-clinton-nancy-reagan-and-aids. Accessed on February 2, 2017.

"Statistics: Worldwide." 2017. amfAR. http://www.amfar. org/worldwide-aids-stats/. Accessed on November 7, 2017.

The STD Project. 2017. "What Is the Difference between HSV1 & HSV2? Oral and Genital Herpes." http://www. thestdproject.com/what-is-the-difference-between-hsv1- hsv2-oral-and-genital-herpes/. Accessed on February 20, 2017.

Stern, Mark Joseph. 2015. "Listen to Reagan's Press Secretary Laugh about Gay People Dying of AIDS." Slate. http:// www.slate.com/blogs/outward/2015/12/01/reagan_press_ secretary_laughs_about_gay_people_dying_of_aids.html. Accessed on February 1, 2017.

Tarnas, Richard. 2011. *The Passion of the Western Mind: Understanding the Ideas That Have Shaped Our World View*. New York: Ballantine Books.

Thomson, Thomas. 1812. *History of the Royal Society, from Its Institution to the End of the Eighteenth Century*. London: Printed for R. Baldwin.

Thorburn, A. L. 1974. "Alfred François Donné, 1801–1878, Discoverer of Trichomonas Vaginalis and of Leukaemia." *British Journal of Venereal Disease*, 50(5): 377–380.

Tidy, Colin. 2014. "Viral Hepatitis (Particularly D and E)." Patient. http://patient.info/doctor/ viral-hepatitis-particularly-d-and-e. Accessed on February 19, 2017.

"Treatment of Syphilis in Early Modern Europe." 2017. Infectious Diseases at the Edward Worth Library. http://infectiousdiseases.edwardworthlibrary.ie/syphilis/treatment/. Accessed on February 10, 2017.

"Vaginal Yeast Infections." 2015. Women's Health. gov. https://www.womenshealth.gov/publications/our-publications/fact-sheet/vaginal-yeast-infections.html?from=AtoZ#. Accessed on February 17, 2017.

Varro, Marcus Terentius. 1934. "On Agriculture." Translated by William Davis Hooper. Cambridge, MA: Harvard University Press. https://babel.hathitrust.org/cgi/pt?id=mdp.39015005105666;view=1up;seq=7. Accessed on December 23, 2017.

Vollmann, Jochen, and Rold Winau. 1996. "Informed Consent in Human Experimentation before the Nuremberg Code." *British Medical Journal,* 313(7070): 1445–1447.

White, Benjamin, and Oswald T. Avery. 1909. "The Treponema Pallidum: Observations on Its Occurrence and Demonstration in Syphilitic Lesions." *Archives of Internal Medicine,* 3(5–6): 411–421.

Willcox, R. R. 1949. "Venereal Disease in the Bible." *The British Journal of Venereal Diseases,* 25(1): 28–33.

Zur Hausen, Harald. 2009. "Papillomaviruses in the Causation of Human Cancers—A Brief Historical Account." *Virology,* 384(2): 260–265.

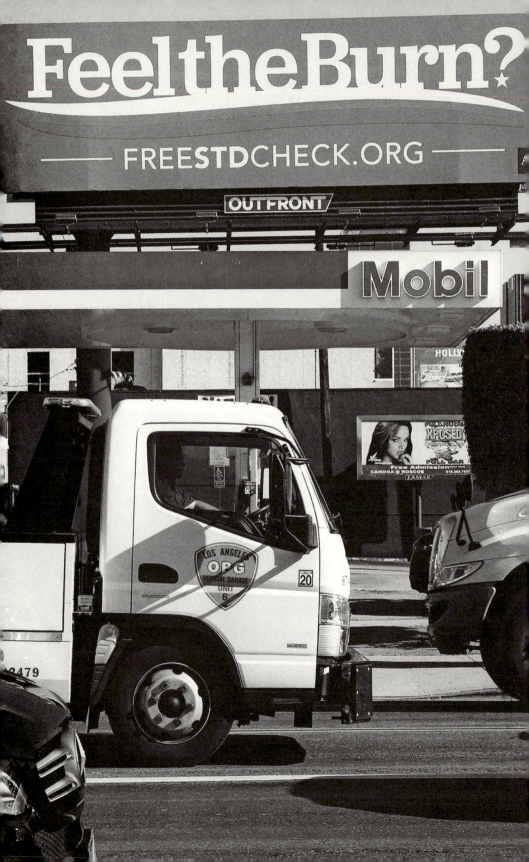

As we approach the end of the 20th century, the United States is faced with a unique opportunity to eliminate syphilis within its borders. Syphilis is easy to detect and cure, given adequate access to and utilization of care. Nationally, it is at the lowest rate ever recorded and it is confined to a very limited number of geographic areas. The last epidemic peaked in 1990, with the highest syphilis rate in 40 years. By 1998, the number of cases had declined by 86 percent. (CDC 1999, 5)

"Cautious Exuberance" to "Troubled Concern"

There was a cautious sense of exuberance in the late 1990s in the United States with regard to the incidence of sexually transmitted infections (STIs) in the country. As the above quotation indicates, perhaps the strongest strain of optimism focused on the possibility that syphilis might actually be eradicated in the nation within the foreseeable future. The U.S. Centers for Disease Control and Prevention (CDC) had actually developed a program "to reduce P&S [primary and secondary] syphilis cases to 1,000 or fewer and to increase the number of syphilis free counties to 90% by 2005" (CDC 1999, 8). As shown in Table 2.1, a rise in the incidence of syphilis cases during the 1980s was followed by a rather dramatic decrease in such cases

---

Billboards like the one shown here are part of an ad campaign by the AIDS Healthcare Foundation, urging anyone who might feel painful symptoms of sexually transmitted diseases to get free screening. (AP Photo/Nick Ut)

Table 2.1   Trends in Incidence of Primary and Secondary Syphilis and
Gonorrhea in the United States, 1978–2000

Year	Primary and Secondary Syphilis		Gonorrhea	
	Cases	Rate[1]	Cases	Rate[1]
1978	21,656	9.8	**1,013,436**	**456.3**
1979	24,874	11.1	1,004,058	447.1
1980	27,204	12.0	1,004,029	442.1
1981	31,266	13.6	990,864	431.8
1982	33,613	14.5	960,633	414.7
1983	32,698	14.0	900,435	385.1
1984	28,607	12.1	878,556	372.5
1985	27,131	11.4	911,419	383.0
1986	27,667	11.5	892,229	371.5
1987	35,585	14.7	787,532	325.0
1988	40,474	16.6	738,160	301.9
1989	45,826	18.6	733,294	297.1
1990	**50,578**	**20.3**	690,042	276.4
1991	42,950	17.0	621,918	245.8
1992	34,009	13.3	502,858	196.0
1993	26,527	10.2	444,649	171.1
1994	20,641	7.8	419,602	163.9
1995	16,543	6.2	392,651	147.5
1996	11,405	4.2	328,169	121.8
1997	8,556	3.1	*327,665*	*120.2*
1998	7,007	2.5	356,492	129.2
1999	6,617	2.4	360,813	129.3
2000	*5,979*	*2.1*	363,136	128.7

Source: Centers for Disease Control and Prevention. 2016. "Sexually Transmitted Diseases—Reported Cases and Rates of Reported Cases per 100,000 Population, United States, 1941–2015." Sexually Transmitted Disease Surveillance 2015, Table 1, pp. 85–86. https://www.cdc.gov/std/stats15/std-surveillance-2015-print.pdf. Accessed on February 10, 2017.

[1]Per 100,000.

Number in bold = Peak year for this time period.

Number in italics = Lowest year for this time period.

during the 1990s. Although less pronounced, a similar pattern was also detectable in the incidence of gonorrhea. Was it possible that these historic scourges of human civilization finally to be brought under control, in at least one part of the world?

As it turned out, the answer to that question was a rather resounding "no." The hopes of the late 1990s for reigning in the horrors of syphilis and gonorrhea were rudely dashed, to be replaced by a somewhat muted sense of impending disaster expressed in formal CDC reports of the mid-2010s. Characteristic of these concerns was the warning issued in the most recent surveillance report on STIs in the United States by Dr. Gail Bolan, director of the CDC's Division of STD Prevention. "Not that long ago," she wrote:

> Gonorrhea rates were at historic lows, syphilis was close to elimination, and we were able to point to advances in STD prevention, such as better chlamydia diagnostic tests and more screening, contributing to increases in detection and treatment of chlamydial infections. That progress has since unraveled. The number of reported syphilis cases is climbing after being largely on the decline since 1941, and gonorrhea rates are now increasing. (Bolan 2015)

The statistical basis for Dr. Bolan's concerns is reflected in the trends shown in Table 2.2.

Table 2.2   Trends in Incidence of Primary and Secondary Syphilis and Gonorrhea in the United States, 2000–2015

Year	Primary and Secondary Syphilis		Gonorrhea	
	Cases	Rate[1]	Cases	Rate[1]
2000	5,979	2.1	363,136	**128.7**
2001	6,103	2.1	361,705	126.8
2002	6,862	2.4	351,852	122.0

(continued)

Table 2.2   (Continued)

Year	Primary and Secondary Syphilis		Gonorrhea	
	Cases	Rate[1]	Cases	Rate[1]
2003	7,177	2.5	335,104	115.2
2004	7,980	2.7	330,132	112.4
2005	8,724	2.9	339,593	114.6
2006	9,756	3.3	358,366	119.7
2007	11,466	3.8	355,991	118.0
2008	13,500	4.4	336,742	110.7
2009	13,997	4.6	*301,174*	*98.1*
2010	13,774	4.5	309,341	100.2
2011	13,970	4.5	321,849	103.3
2012	15,667	5.0	334,826	106.7
2013	17,375	5.5	333,004	105.3
2014	19,999	6.3	350,062	109.8
2015	**23,872**	**7.5**	**395,216**	123.9

Source: Centers for Disease Control and Prevention. 2016. "Sexually Transmitted Diseases—Reported Cases and Rates of Reported Cases per 100,000 Population, United States, 1941–2015." Sexually Transmitted Disease Surveillance 2015, Table 1, pp. 85–86. https://www.cdc.gov/std/stats15/std-surveillance-2015-print. pdf. Accessed on February 10, 2017.

[1]Per 100,000.

Number in bold = Peak year for this time period.

Number in italics = Lowest year for this time period.

So what went wrong in the United States between 1999 and 2015? What factors are responsible in the reappearance of STIs as major public health issues of concern today? No simple, single answer is available for that question. Instead, a confluence of factors has led from the "cautious exuberance" of the late 1990s to a more "troubled concern" of the mid-2010s.

The Battle against Gonorrhea

In some cases, technical challenges confronting researchers at least partially explain the increase in STI rates. Gonorrhea was perhaps the best example. Prior to the 1930s, researchers had tried a host of natural products and synthetic drugs for the treatment of gonorrhea. In the decades preceding and following the turn of the 20th century, the most popular forms of treatment for gonorrhea were two natural products: cubebs, a type of pepper grown in Indonesia, and a resin of the copaiba tree (*Copaifera officinalis*) that grows primarily in South America. During the early 1900s, researchers turned to a variety of inorganic heavy metal compounds, including arsenic, antimony, bismuth, gold, and mercury (Benedek n.d.). These materials were only partially successful, at best, in curing the disease. And it was not until the 1930s that a truly effective curative agent became available: the sulfonamides.

In the late 1920 and early 1930s, German pathologist Gerhard Domagk discovered that a class of chemical compounds known as the sulfonamides (or "sulfa drugs") were effective in killing, among other pathogens, the bacterium responsible for gonorrhea, *Neisseria gonorrhoeae*. Many workers were elated with what they believed might be the "magic bullet" against gonorrhea. Data collected about the use of the sulfonamides for the treating of wounds only seemed to confirm the promise of the compounds for the treatment of infectious diseases.

It was not long, however, before medical workers began to recognize a phenomenon that was later to become a crucial aspect of all forms of disease treatment: the development of resistance to a drug. It is now well known that microorganisms mutate and evolve over time in such a way as to become less susceptible and more resistant to any given chemical substance to which they are exposed. Such proved to be the case with the first commercially available sulfonamide, Prontosil. Within a decade of its introduction, Prontosil's efficacy in the treatment of gonorrhea began to decrease. Researchers' response to this phenomenon caused them to look for other types of sulfonamides, with more than 5,000 such compounds eventually having been tested for treatment against gonorrhea and other infectious diseases (Van Miert 1994).

By the mid-1940s, clinicians began to switch over from the sulfanilamides to the next "wonder drug," penicillin. That drug continued to be the treatment of choice for nearly four decades, being supplemented in 1949 with another new antibiotic, tetracycline. By the late 1980s, both penicillin and tetracycline had essentially lost their effectiveness against *N. gonorrhoeae* and were replaced in the 1990s, once again, by another class of antibiotics, the fluoroquinolones, which held their place in treatment systems for little more than a decade. In 2007, the CDC recommended discontinuing the use of fluoroquinolones for the treatment of gonorrhea, and replacing them with yet another class of compounds, the cephalosporins. Three years later, the CDC changed its recommendations once more, moving to a combination therapy for gonorrhea consisting of a cephalosporin (ceftriaxone or cefixime) given by injection plus either azithromycin or doxycycline orally (Del Rio et al. 2012). In its 2015 report on STIs, the CDC announced that questions were being raised as to whether even this "treatment of last resort" was likely to be effective much longer.

How did this new threat to the treatment of gonorrhea develop? Current research now suggests that this phenomenon may have had its start in Japan during the 1990s when one of the drugs used for the treatment of gonorrhea, ceftriaxone, was no longer used by medical workers. In addition, lower doses of the other effective drug, cefixime, were used for treatment. The combination of these actions apparently increased the ability of *N. gonorrhoeae* to adapt to the two drugs and develop resistance to them. In a world in which widespread travel is common, then, the drug-resistant strains of the agent began to spread to nearby countries, such as Australia, China, Hong Kong, and Taiwan, and, eventually throughout the world (Unemo and Nicholas 2012). A turning point of sorts was reached in 2013 when the first cases of nontreatable gonorrhea were reported in North America. Of 133 patients with gonorrhea treated by current conventional therapy, 9 were found to have retained *N. gonorrhoeae* within their bodies; that is, treatment had been a failure. All nine patients were eventually cured by injections of high-dose drugs, but any barrier that may have existed protecting the continent from drug-resistant gonorrhea had obviously been breached (Allen et al. 2013).

Perhaps the more important question is what can be done to deal with gonococcal infections now that existing medicinal options have been so drastically reduced. One answer is obviously to take two steps: increase the dosage and find more effective ways of using drugs that are still effective against *N. gonorrhoeae* and accelerate the search for new drugs that are effective against the pathogen. Somewhat desperate for a solution to this problem, researchers are now pursuing both of these objectives.

The search for new anti-infective agents has already produced some promising candidates. Researchers at Massachusetts-based Entasis Therapeutics reported in late 2015 on the early success of drug designated as ETX0914 (formerly AZD0914) in the treatment of gonorrhea (Entasis Therapeutics 2017). A CDC research team also reported in 2013 on a dual therapeutic regimen consisting of an injection of gentamicin plus azithromycin delivered orally, or a combination of gemifloxacin plus azithromycin, delivered orally (Kirkcaldy 2013).

The problem with this technological approach, of course, is that one can predict that any new drug, combination of drugs, or dosage pattern will be effective for only a limited period of time. History has shown that pathogens evolve to become to resistant to essentially any drug developed for their treatment. In this respect, it has become necessary and popular among specialists in STI prevention and treatment to think of approaches other than the development of new drugs. This approach has been perhaps best illustrated by a document issued in 2012 by the World Health Organization (WHO), "Global Action Plan to Control the Spread and Impact of Antimicrobial Resistance in *Neisseria gonorrhoeae*" (WHO 2012). That document emphasizes the importance of supplementing research on new drugs with an enhanced program of public education to inform people about the nature of gonorrhea, the risks it poses to a person's health, the means of transmission, and the steps that can be taken to prevent infection by the *N. gonorrhoeae* bacterium.

The eight strategies outlined by the WHO document are as follows:

1. Advocacy for increased awareness on correct use of antibiotics among health care providers and the consumer, particularly in key populations including men who have sex with men (MSM) and sex workers

2. Effective prevention, diagnosis, and control of gonococcal infections, using prevention messages and prevention interventions, and recommended adequate diagnosis and appropriate treatment regimens

3. Systematic monitoring of treatment failures by developing a standard case definition of treatment failure, and protocols for verification, reporting and management of treatment failure

4. Effective drug regulations and prescription policies

5. Strengthened antimicrobial resistance surveillance, especially in countries with a high burden of gonococcal infections, other STIs, and human immunodeficiency virus (HIV)

6. Capacity building to establish regional networks of laboratories to perform gonococcal culture, with good-quality control mechanisms

7. Research into newer molecular methods for monitoring and detecting antimicrobial resistance

8. Research into, and identification of, alternative effective treatment regimens for gonococcal infections (WHO 2012, 5)

The document then goes on to describe in detail the specific actions that can be taken by various stakeholders to achieve these objectives. It points out that the battle against *N. gonorrhoeae* requires the coordinated efforts of a wide variety of organizations, including WHO itself, ministries of health and STI agencies, donor organizations, national public health laboratories, the private sector and nongovernmental organizations, clinicians, and researchers. Among the activities in which these groups must be involved are basic and applied research, creation of supportive policies, establishment of norms for testing and prevention, surveillance of incidence and prevalence, advocacy and public engagement, drug regulation, creation and maintenance of early warning systems for gonorrheal outbreaks, and communication and education, especially among populations at special risk for the disease (WHO 2012, 5–7).

One of the overriding issues at the base of current gonorrheal problems is the simple fact of funding. At the very time that medical treatment for the disease has become less effective, funding agencies have, for a variety of reasons, either maintained existing budgets for research, education, prevention, and treatment or, in many cases, actually cut back on funding. Some commentators have noted that the slowdown and/or cutbacks in funding for STIs was probably influenced to some extent by the financial crisis that swept the United States and other parts of the world in 2008 (National Coalition of STD Directors 2016). In the United States, for example, the U.S. Congress has maintained funding for STI programs at a fairly constant level over the past decade. During that time, funding for STI activities within the National Institute of Allergy and Infectious Disease has hovered around $4.5 billion annually, reaching a high of $4,977,070,000 in 2011 and a low of $4,423,357,000 in 2015 (National Institute of Allergy and Infectious Diseases 2016, 8). Funding for programs in HIV, viral hepatitis, STIs, and TB have also remained relatively stable between 2012 and 2015 at about $1.1 billion (Department of Health and Human Services 2016a, 69).

The impact of the recession on state and local programs for STI was probably worse than even at the federal level.

According to a presentation made by Gail Bolan, director of the CDC Division of STD Prevention, 52 percent of local health departments (LHDs) reported experiencing budget cuts in 2012. The most common cutbacks involved reduced hours (42.8% of LHDs); reduced screening (40.0%); reduced contact tracing for chlamydia, gonorrhea, and other nonsyphilis infections; increases in fees or co-pays (33.9%); and outright closures (6.8%). Overall, an estimated 21 LHDs simply closed their STI clinics entirely.

Another factor impacting the amount of money that governments spend on STIs is that cutbacks in some programs unrelated to STIs may, in fact, have unintended consequences for STI programs. For example, the Republican Party in the United States has for some time objected to the use of federal funds to support programs by the organization known as Planned Parenthood. The argument was that the organization provides abortions for women, a policy to which the GOP is opposed. Soon after Republicans gained power in the U.S. Congress and the Executive Office in January 2017, members of the administration and legislature, acting on this position, began actions to defund Planned Parenthood. In its program to eliminate the Affordable Care Act of 2010, for example, the Republican majority in the U.S. Congress voted to end all funding for Planned Parenthood programs (Crockett 2017).

The problem with this approach for health care workers is that Planned Parenthood spends by far the greatest portion of its budget (45%) on STI/STD testing and treatment, followed by contraception programs (31%), other women's health services (13%), and cancer screening and prevention (7%). A paltry 3 percent goes to abortion services. Thus, defunding the organization, however one may feel about the issue of abortion, has a far more serious effect on the 4,218,149 visits relating to STD/STI issues than it does on the 323,999 visits for abortion services (Planned Parenthood 2015).

One hope for the ongoing problem of gonorrheal infections is the development of a vaccine to provide protection against infection. As of 2017, no vaccine is available for any of the bacterial STIs, including gonorrhea, although research continues on such technologies in a variety of laboratories. One challenge in the development of a gonorrheal vaccine is the rapid mutation of antigens on the surface of the bacterium that makes it difficult to produce a vaccine with ongoing effectiveness. Also, until very recently, there have been no animal models on which vaccines could be tested.

Some breakthroughs have recently been announced, however. For example, in 2013, a research team led by immunologist Michael W. Russell at the University at Buffalo of the State University of New York found that the insertion of a time-release nanoparticle-based drug originally developed for the treatment of cancer showed promise in inducing long-term resistance in experimental mice to infection by *N. gonorrhoeae*. The researchers concluded that their research "may serve as novel, safe approaches to the treatment and prevention of this very common sexually transmitted infection" (Liu, Egilmez, and Russell 2013; also see Jerse, Bash, and Russell 2014).

Syphilis: A Disheartening State of Affairs

An editorial in the June 7, 2016, issue of *JAMA* (*The Journal of the American Medical Association*) reviewed the status of the incidence of syphilis in the United States (Clement and Hicks 2016). It began with a reminder of the optimistic outlook in the fight against the disease reflected in the CDC's 1999 National Plan to Eliminate Syphilis in the United States cited at the beginning of this chapter. The CDC then went on to say that, as of 2016, "hopes for eradication have long since faded" (Clement and Hicks 2016, 2281).

The trend in new primary and secondary cases shown in Tables 2.1 and 2.2 is puzzling, to begin with, because the 1999 plan to eliminate the diseases was based on sound scientific and medical evidence. In the first place, the efficacy of tests for the detection and diagnosis of all stages of syphilis has been and continues to be very high: 78–86 percent for primary syphilis, 100 percent for secondary syphilis, and 96–98 percent for latent syphilis (Bibbins-Domingo et al. 2016, 2325; this document is often referred to by the acronym USPSTF). These numbers suggest that individuals who present at clinics with possible symptoms of the disease can learn of their status with a very high degree of confidence. In addition, treatment for the disease is also very reliable. The most recent CDC guidelines for treatment of STIs, for example, note that:

> The effectiveness of penicillin for the treatment of syphilis was well established through clinical experience even before the value of randomized controlled clinical trials was recognized. Therefore, nearly all recommendations for the treatment of syphilis are based not only on clinical trials and observational studies, but many decades of clinical experience. (Workowski and Bolan 2015)

(A single dose of 2.4 million units of benzathine penicillin G administered intramuscularly is now the recommended treatment for all stages of the disease in adults and 50,000 units per kilogram of body weight for children [Workowski and Bolan 2015].)

In its review of syphilis treatment, the USPSTF also included an assessment of potential risks to individuals who might be tested and treated for syphilis. The USPSTF concluded that such individuals among men and nonpregnant women posed no significant harm, such as "possible false-positive results that require clinical evaluation, unnecessary anxiety to the patient, and the potential stigma of having a sexually transmitted infection" (Bibbins-Domingo et al. 2016, 2322). The task force came to the conclusion that "with high certainty . . . the net benefit of screening for syphilis infection in nonpregnant persons at increased risk for infection is substantial" (Bibbins-Domingo et al. 2016, 2323).

Given this optimistic view of the current status of diagnosis and treatment for syphilis, the fundamental question remains, to quote a major analysis of the problem, "what went wrong?" between 1999 and 2016. The authors of this analysis focus on three events and conditions that may explain the nation's setback in its battle against syphilis. The first problem is one that has been discussed above: reductions in the funds available to conduct adequate education, prevention, treatment, and research programs on the control of syphilis. Federal funding for all STI programs has remained relatively constant over the past five years, as shown in Table 2.3. Supporters of strong syphilis reduction programs argue that decreasing funds for prevention and treatment programs at a time when infections are increasing is not good policy. They point to studies that show that modest investments in prevention programs can result in significant long-term savings in treatment programs. One such study, for example, found that every ten cents per capita invested in prevention programs resulted in a 30 percent decrease in the rate of early syphilis for targeted populations (National Coalition of STD Directors n.d.).

Table 2.3   Funding for STD Prevention Programs, 2012–2017

Fiscal Year	Appropriation (in millions)
2012	$163
2013	$154.9
2014	$157.7
2015	$157.3
2016	$157.3
2017	$157.3

Sources: National Coalition of STD Directors. 2015. "Support FY 2016 STD Prevention Funding." http://federalaidspolicy.org/wp-content/uploads/2015/04/FINAL-FY16-Support-STD-Prevention-Funding.pdf. Accessed on February 13, 2017. Centers for Disease Control and Prevention. 2016. "Overview of Budget Request," 1. https://www.cdc.gov/budget/documents/fy2017/fy-2017-cdc-budget-overview.pdf. Accessed on February 13, 2017.

Such arguments appear not to have much appeal to legislators who control the purse strings for STI funding at the federal level. For example, even in light of the growing STI problems in the United States, the Senate Appropriations Committee in October 2016 voted to *decrease* funding for such programs by about $5 million, or about 3 percent, for FY2017. The Congress as a whole later defeated that recommendation and kept STI funding at the same level as for 2015 and 2016 (CDC 2016g, 1).

Another factor that appears to be affecting the incidence of primary and secondary syphilis in the United States (and in Western Europe, as well) is a rapid rise in the number of cases of the infection among MSM The term is now much preferred over earlier categories such as "gay men" and "bisexual men" because it focuses on the mechanism by which a specific disease is transmitted and the burden of that infection in society, rather than on a person's sexual orientation ("gay," "straight," "bisexual," "pansexual," etc.). A similar term is used for women who have sex with women, WSW (Vanderbuilt University 2017).

At the annual CDC STD Prevention Conference held in Atlanta in 2016, one group of researchers reported that 81.7 percent of all new primary and secondary syphilis cases for which partners could be identified occurred among MSM (CDC 2017d). This number continued a trend dating back to the early 2000s during which MSM have continued to provide a significantly greater proportion of new syphilis cases compared to the numbers in the overall society (CDC 2016j, 77).

The explanation for this trend is relatively easy to discern. During the late 1980s and 1990s, the rise of HIV/AIDS within the gay community dramatically increased the awareness of gay men of the risks of having unprotected sex. As a result, most gay men and other MSM began to take a number of measures to protect themselves from HIV infection, including the use of condoms, greatly reduced attendance at locations where transmission was likely to occur (such as gay bathhouses), and the pursuit of fewer sexual partners (Whittington et al. 2002, 1010). Coincidentally, these actions also decreased the risk of contracting other STIs through casual, unprotected sex (O'Leary 2014).

Progress in programs for the prevention and treatment of HIV that came online during the early 2000s changed this trend. As HIV infection no longer became a "death sentence," many MSM individuals decided to neglect some of the highly effective infection-preventative methods that they had adopted only a few years earlier. Such behaviors increased the risk not only for HIV (which, at least now could be kept under control by new retroviral medications), but also for other STIs, such as syphilis (Clement and Hicks 2016, 2282; Truong et al. 2006).

Programs of prevention and treatment for MSM present special challenges for public health programs. Members of this population often face problems with access to such programs not experienced by heterosexual males and females not only because of their sexual choices, but also because they may belong to a racial, ethnic, economic, or other minority. Searching for ways to overcome these barriers to medical assistance for STI-related problems is a growing challenge, therefore, for public health workers (McKirnan et al. 2013; for a detailed discussion of this issue, also see Workowski and Bolan 2015).

Yet another factor in the rise of syphilis rates in the general population, and among MSM in particular, may have been the emphasis placed on HIV issues in the United States beginning in the late 1980s. Total federal expenditures on HIV/AIDS-related problems amounted to less than $500 million from the disease's first appearance in 1981 to 1988. As Table 2.4 shows, the total annual budget for the CDC in 1984 was about $215 million, compared to an expenditure of about $44 million for all HIV/AIDS research. Federal HIV/AIDS expenditures then began to rise rapidly, generally at a rate of 10–35 percent per year, depending on the specific program involved. As Table 2.4 shows, federal funding for HIV/AIDS programs had reached $18.5 billion by 2004. At the same time, federal funding for

Table 2.4   Federal Funding, All Disease Control, Research and Training
(from CDC) versus All Federal Funding for HIV/AIDS, 1984–2004
(in billions of dollars)

Year	All CDC[1]	All HIV/AIDS[2]
1984[3]	$0.215	$0.044
1997	$2.302	$8.8
1998	$2.383	$9.7
1999	$2.609	$10.8
2000	$2.962	$12.2
2001	$3.868	$14.4
2002	$4.293	$15.2
2003	$4.296	$16.8
2004	$4.367	$18.5

Sources: Centers for Disease Control and Prevention. Department of Health and Human Services Fiscal Year 2006. Justification of Estimates for Appropriation Committees. https://www.cdc.gov/budget/documents/fy2006/fy-2006-cdc-congressional-justification.pdf. Accessed on February 14, 2017; Summers, Todd, and Jennifer Kates. 2004. "Trends in U.S. Government Funding for HIV/AIDS, Fiscal Years 1981–2004." The Henry J. Kaiser Family Foundation. https://kaiserfamilyfoundation.files.wordpress.com/2013/01/issue-brief-trends-in-u-s-government-funding-for-hiv-aids-fiscal-years-1981-to-2004.pdf. Accessed on February 14, 2017, Figure 2, page 2.

For FY1984 only: National Center for Biotechnology Information. 1991. "Supporting the NIH AIDS Research Program." The AIDS Research Program of the National Institutes of Health. https://www.ncbi.nlm.nih.gov/books/NBK234085/. Accessed on February 15, 2017; "Budget of the United States Government Fiscal Year 1984." 1984. Fraser. https://fraser.stlouisfed.org/scribd/?item_id=18990&filepath=/files/docs/publications/usbudget/bus_1984.pdf, 8-86. Accessed on February 15, 2017.

[1] Appropriation.

[2] Expenditure.

[3] For comparison.

all STI programs remained relatively constant. These patterns reflect the realization by legislators over time that the HIV epidemic was serious, it was growing, and research on the disease required significant financial support. Thus, between 1997 and 2004, funding for HIV/AIDS programs increased by more than 110 percent, while funding for all CDC programs grew by only 89 percent. That pattern continues to hold true today, with the fiscal year 2016 budget allotting $11.5 billion to all CDC expenses and $27.4 billion to all HIV/AIDS programs (Department of Health and Human Services 2017; Henry J. Kaiser Family Foundation 2016). What these figures suggest is that (the very legitimate) concerns about perhaps the most serious of all STIs during the past few decades, HIV, has "drained off" federal funds that might otherwise have gone to STI programs (see also Clement and Hicks 2016, 2282).

A New Kind of Challenge: Chlamydia

Students of STIs often focus their attention on two of the oldest and best-known diseases: syphilis and gonorrhea. One reason for this pattern is that both diseases have been around for at least two thousand years, and, if left untreated, they both can have dire consequences for someone who is infected with their causative agents. Yet, there is a third STI that, in terms of numbers alone, dwarfs the significance of both syphilis and gonorrhea: chlamydia. According to the most recent data available, 1,526,658 cases of the infection were reported in the United States in 2015, making its rate 478.8 cases per 100,000 Americans. To appreciate the simple magnitude of the chlamydia problem, compare those numbers with the incidence of primary and secondary syphilis in the same year (23,872; 7.5) and gonorrhea (395,216; 123.9). The severity of the chlamydia problem is also reflected in the fact that the disease was not even a required reportable disease until 1984, when 7,594 cases of the infection were recorded, compared to 28,607 cases of syphilis and 878,556 cases of gonorrhea in the same year (CDC 2016i). Global statistics are similar to those for the United States. A 2016 WHO report estimated that 131 million new cases of chlamydia are reported every year, making it the most common STI in terms of numbers of all such infections (WHO 2016b).

Chlamydia is an STI caused by the bacterium *Chlamydia trachomatis*. It may cause cervicitis (inflammation of the cervix) in women and urethritis (inflammation of the urethra) and proctitis (inflammation of the lining of the rectum) in both men and women. Although the disease is not fatal, it can, if left untreated, lead to a number of other health conditions for women later in life, such as infertility, ectopic pregnancy, chronic pelvic pain, pregnancy complications, and pelvic inflammatory disease (PID), which may itself lead to other more serious health problems. In men, untreated chlamydial infections can result in epididymitis (inflammation of the testicles) and nonreactive arthritis (inflammation of connective tissue; National Health Service [UK] 2015).

Chlamydia can be transmitted by any mechanism involved in sexual intercourse, at the mouth, penis, vagina, or anus. A woman who is infected with chlamydia can also transmit the disease to her newborn child during delivery. The incubation period for chlamydia is not known precisely, but is thought to be of the order of a few weeks.

A large fraction of chlamydial infections remain asymptomatic; that is, a person does not know that he or she has been infected. A number of studies have been done on specific groups of individuals to find the rate at which symptoms appear, but they are much lower than for most any other form of STI. By one estimate, no more than 10 percent of men and between 5 and 30 percent of women do develop signs and symptoms of the disease (CDC 2016c; Detels et al. 2011).

The asymptomatic character of chlamydia accounts for one of the most challenging problems involved in dealing with the infection. A person infected with *Treponema pallidum* or *N. gonorrhoeae* normally has clear signs and symptoms of the disease that cause him or her to become concerned and to seek medical attention. For example, suppose that a young man suddenly notices the presence of a milky white discharge from his penis, accompanied by pain during urination. It will probably be difficult for that individual to just ignore the condition. Instead, he is likely to go to his own physician or a public health clinic to get advice about the problem. In turn, the doctor or public health worker will conduct a test to determine whether the individual actually has an STI.

But the situation with chlamydia is different. The majority—perhaps the vast majority—of women and men infected with *C. trachomatis* will not experience *any* signs or symptoms of the disease. They will go on with their lives in a normal fashion, which may include sexual contact with other individuals, resulting in an ever-widening circle of infections.

For this reason, health officials generally emphasize the importance of *screening* programs for the control of chlamydia infections, rather than depending on *testing* for the disease. These two diagnostic techniques differ from each other in the following way: a person who suspects, or whose health care worker suspects, that he or she may have an infection of some type can request or have ordered a standard test for determining the presence of an infectious agent. For example, tests are available to determine whether a person has been infected with the *T. pallidum* bacterium. By contrast, screening programs test a wide population of individuals for a disease, whether or not they have signs or symptoms of an infection. This approach allows health care workers to determine if a person is infected with a causative agent, even when he or she does not suspect that such may be the case.

In actual practice, there are a number of differences between screening and testing procedures, above and beyond the description provided thus far. For example, since screening programs are designed to reach a wide population of individuals, they need to be relatively simple and inexpensive to perform. By contrast, because of the high likelihood that an infection exists, testing programs can be more complex and more expensive. In addition, the participants in a screening program need to be convinced of the importance of the program and be willing to volunteer in being examined. In testing programs, a person probably already has a strong suspicion that his or her health has been compromised and may be more willing and eager to be tested. In some circumstances, when public health is an issue, individuals suspected of having an STI may be *required* to have a test for the disease (Ruf and Morgan 2008). Current CDC recommendations for the screening for chlamydia are given in Table 2.5.

One of the procedures recommended in Table 2.5, test-of-cure, may need further definition. With the treatment for any STI, it is important to make sure that the treatment provided

Table 2.5   Current Screening Recommendations for Chlamydia

Population	Recommended Screening
Women	• Sexually active women under 25 years of age • Sexually active women aged 25 years and older if at increased risk[1] • Retest approximately 3 months after treatment
Pregnant Women	• All pregnant women under 25 years of age • Pregnant women, aged 25 and older if at increased risk[1] • Retest during the 3rd trimester for women under 25 years of age or at risk • Pregnant women with chlamydial infection should have a test-of-cure 3–4 weeks after treatment and be retested within 3 months
Men	• Consider screening young men in high prevalence clinical settings, such as adolescent clinics, correctional facilities, and STD clinics, or in populations with high burden of infection, such as MSM
MSM	• At least annually for sexually active MSM at sites of contact (urethra, rectum) regardless of condom use • Every 3–6 months if at increased risk[2]
Persons with HIV	• For sexually active individuals, screen at first HIV evaluation, and at least annually thereafter • More frequent screening might be appropriate depending on individual risk behaviors and the local epidemiology

Source: Centers for Disease Control and Prevention. 2016. "Screening Recommendations and Considerations Referenced in Treatment Guidelines and Original Sources." https://www.cdc.gov/std/tg2015/screening-recommendations.htm. Accessed on February 16, 2017.

[1]Those who have a new sex partner, more than one sex partner, a sex partner with concurrent partners, or a sex partner who has an STI.

[2]Those with HIV infection if risk behaviors persist or if they or their sexual partners have multiple partners.

for that disease has actually been infected in destroying the causative agent. With syphilis and gonorrhea, a test-of-cure is generally not necessary since a person will know if his or her signs and symptoms reoccur. With chlamydia, that is not the case. If treatment fails, a person may be asymptomatic and, therefore, not aware that the treatment has been unsuccessful. A test-of-cure procedure simply involves the retest of an individual who has been treated to the disease, to make sure that it has actually been cured. (It should be noted, however, that some question has been raised as to the actual effectiveness of current test-of-cure procedures; see, for example, Dukers-Muijrers et al. 2012.)

Chlamydia infections are sometimes confused with another type of disease affecting the genital area, a yeast infection. Most yeast infections are caused by a type of fungus called *Candida albicans*. The organism occurs naturally in a woman's vagina and poses no health issues for her. From time to time, however, the amount of *C. albicans* present may increase significantly, resulting in a yeast infection. Experts believe that up to 75 percent of all women will have a yeast infection at some time in their lives.

Yeast infections are not considered to be STIs since they are not generally a result of sexual activities. They are characterized by an itchiness or burning of the vagina, accompanied by burning during urination. They may also be apparent because of a milky white discharge that may be either clear or thick. Yeast infections are easily cured by application of an over-the-counter antifungal cream, ointment, tablet, or suppository, such as butoconazole (Gynazole), miconazole (Lotrimin), and terconazole (Terazol). A single dose of an oral medication, such as fluconazole (Diflucan), is also effective.

Yeast infections may also occur in men, although such events are quite rare. They occur when a man has sexual intercourse with a woman who has a yeast infection. As with women, yeast infections in men can be cured relatively easily and seldom lead to more serious health problems (Thaler 2015).

A Harbinger of Cancer: Pelvic Inflammatory Disease

PID is an infection of the upper part of the female reproductive system, including the uterus, ovaries, and fallopian tubes. It is caused by any number of bacteria, most prominently *C. trachomatis* and *N. gonorrhoeae*, but also including *Streptococcus pyogenes*, *Gardnerella vaginalis*, *Escherichia coli*, and *Bacteroides* spp. Thus, while the vast majority of PID cases occur as the result of sexual interactions with an affected person, the disease may also develop for reasons other than such activity (Sharma et al. 2014).

PID has been known and studied (although not always under that name) for more than 500 years. One of the first formal descriptions was written by the French physician François Mauriceau, who wrote about its symptoms in his 1683 work, *Traite Des Maladies Des Femmes Grosses* (*On the Treatment of Diseases of Large Women*; Viborga 2006). Today the incidence of PID in the American population is thought to be about 4.4 percent among sexually experienced reproductive-aged woman, an estimate that equates to about 2.5 million women in the country with the disease in 2014 (Kreisel et al. 2017).

Both men and women may experience PID, although the condition is much more common in women than in men. A person with the infection may be asymptomatic or may experience signs and symptoms that they do not associate with the disease, such as dysuria (pain with urination), dyspareunia (pain with sexual intercourse), or gastrointestinal symptoms. Other common symptoms include lower abdominal or pelvic pain, cramping, post-coital vaginal bleeding, vaginal discharge, and fever. Serious consequences of PID infection may include chronic pelvic pain, ectopic pregnancy, and infertility. The most serious complication of PID infections has for some time thought to be increased risk for cervical cancer.

At one time, less than half a century ago, cervical cancer was the leading cause of death among women in the United States.

That situation has changed over the past few decades in this country largely because of increased methods of diagnosis and treatment. In 2013, the most recent year for which data are available, 11,955 women were diagnosed with cervical cancer in the United States, and 4,217 died of the disease, an incidence rate of 8.1 percent (CDC 2016b). The disease is still a matter of major concern worldwide where an estimate 528,000 new cases are observed each year, with a mortality of 266,000 annually. The disease is especially common in parts of Africa, where the incidence rate ranges from 75.9 percent in Malawi and 65.0 percent in Mozambique to 38.4 percent in Guinea in Lesotho (Globocan 2015; World Cancer Research Fund International 2015).

Cervical cancer is caused by a pathogen known as the *human papillomavirus* (HPV). That term applies to more than 170 types of viruses, of which about 40 may infect the human genital tract (Hahn and Spach 2017). Each virus is given its own characteristic designation, such as HPV 16, HPV 18, and HPV 66 (Schoenstadt 2017). HPV may infect both men and women, and is transmitted most often by some form of sexual contact. Recent studies in the United States have shown that nearly half of all Americans are now infected by strains of the virus that occur in the genital region (McQuillan et al. 2017; see Table 5.7 in Chapter 5).

The various types of HPV are generally classified into two categories: low-risk nononcongenic (noncancer-causing) and high-risk oncogenic (cancer-causing) viruses. One very common type of STI, genital warts, is caused by HPV6 and HPV11. For the most parts, however, low-risk viruses cause no serious problems and resolve on their own within a period of about two years. The high risk viruses HPV16 and HPV18 are now thought to account for about 63 percent of all cervical cancers, while HPV types 31, 33, 45, 52, and 58 are considered to be responsible for a variety of other cancers (Hahn and Spach 2017). A commonly quoted statistic is that the family of HPV viruses is responsible for 99 percent of all cervical tumors (Newson 2015).

The incidence of cervical cancer (and many other countries) has shown a significant decline over the past 40 years. Between 1975 and 1982, the annual percentage decrease was 4.3 percent, followed by an annual percentage change of –1.6 percent between 1982 and 1996, –3.8 percent between 1996 and 2003, and –0.9 percent between 2003 and 2012 (Ryerson et al. 2016, Table 1). Health authorities attribute this decline to improved methods of diagnosis and better education for women that encourages them to obtain regular screening, such as so-called pap tests, for the disease (National Institutes of Health 2013).

An important new weapon was added to the battle against HPV infections, and thus cervical cancer, in 2006 with the release of a new vaccine for the infection. Research on the vaccine had begun as early as 1982, when a link between HPVs and various forms of cancer had been definitely demonstrated (Zur Hausen 2009). More than two decades later, a vaccine called Gardasil had been produced that was both safe and efficacious against HPV infections. It was approved by the U.S. Food and Drug Administration (FDA) with the observation that "Today is an important day for public health and for women's health and for our continued fight against serious life-threatening diseases like cervical cancer" (U.S. Food and Drug Administration 2016). In October 2009, the FDA approved a second HPV vaccine called Cervarix, and in 2014, a third such vaccine, Gardasil 9. In August 2016, it announced that it would no longer market Cervarix in the U.S. market, although it would continue to sell the product in other parts of the world. That decision left Merck, as the sole producer of HPV vaccines (Gardasil and Gardasil 9) in the United States (Sagonowsky 2016).

The availability of a vaccine that would protect women against cervical cancer at first seemed like an exciting breakthrough in treatment technologies for STIs. Only a year after the introduction of Gardasil to the marketplace, the American Academy of Pediatricians (AAP) issued a position statement recommending that vaccine for females as young as 11 years of age (Committee on Infectious Diseases 2007). In 2011, AAP extended that recommendation to include boys (Committee on Infectious Diseases 2012; the AAP's current recommendations for vaccinations are available at https://www.cdc.gov/vaccines/schedules/downloads/child/0-18yrs-child-combined-schedule.pdf). Other health groups, such as the American Academy of Family Physicians, American College of Obstetricians and Gynecologists, American College of Physicians, the CDC, and the Immunization Action Coalition, have echoed the original AAP recommendations (Immunization Action Coalition 2016).

Possibly influenced by the position of these important health groups, a number of states began considering legislation that would require (1) schools to provide information about HPV, (2) health insurance companies to pay the cost of HPV vaccination, and/or (3) students to be vaccinated with the HPV vaccine prior to entering elementary or middle school. During the 2006–2007 school year, legislators in 41 states and the District of Columbia considered bills on one or more of these requirements. Of the many bills considered during that period, eight passed: two that would require HPV vaccination as a condition for entering public school (District of Columbia and Virginia), two that required the state department of health to provide information about HPV and the vaccine (North Carolina and Washington), one that provided funding for educational materials about the disease and vaccine (North Dakota), one that would require insurers to pay the cost of HPV vaccinations (Rhode Island), one that provided funding for HPV vaccinations for those between the ages of 11 and 18 who requested it (South Dakota), and one that created an educational campaign about cervical cancer (Utah). Interest in HPV legislation dropped off after 2007, however, with about a dozen states considering legislation on the topic each school year since then. In the school year 2015–2016, for example, 10 states considered a total of 23 different bills (National Conference of State Legislators 2017). The most controversial legislation relating to the HPV vaccine has been the school mandate provision which would require that students be vaccinated against the HPV prior to enrolling in a public school. A number of efforts have been made to remove this requirement in the state of Virginia, all of which have failed. The only additional state that has adopted this requirement since 2007 is Rhode Island, which took this action in 2015, not through the legislative process, but by adding it to the state's department of health school-entering provisions.

Probably the most widely discussed of the school mandate provisions was the executive order issued by Governor Rick Perry, of Texas, on February 2, 2007. Essentially repeating the arguments for required vaccination presented by the APA and other organizations, Perry ordered that "the Health and Human Services Executive Commissioner shall adopt rules that mandate the age appropriate vaccination of all female children for HPV prior to admission to the sixth grade." In addition, he ordered that the state assume the financial costs of carrying out this mandate (Executive Order RP65 2007).

Perry's action set off a brouhaha that spread throughout the state and, before long, across the nation. The Texas legislature took a very different view of the executive order and, on May 8, 2007, passed HB 1098, rescinding the governor's dictate. The governor let the bill become law without his signature and made an extended speech in which he reiterated the basis for his decision and his dissatisfaction with the legislature's action (Perry 2007). Interestingly enough, Perry's position on HPV vaccination later came back to haunt him when he ran for the Republican nomination for president of the United States in 2011. In a now-famous debate during that campaign, another candidate, Michele Bachmann (R-MN), argued that the HPV vaccine could cause mental retardation and that Perry had acted improperly by issuing his executive order on the vaccine. By that time, however, Perry had long previously admitted that he had not considered this problem and should have submitted his HPV plan to the legislature rather than issuing an executive order (Farley 2011).

The HPV vaccine would appear to be an important new tool in the prevention of one of the most serious diseases affecting women: cervical cancer. Yet, more than a decade after the vaccine became available, its use has lagged far beyond the federal government's goal of having at least 80 percent of females between the ages of 13 and 15 receive three doses of the vaccine (HealthyPeople.gov 2017b, IID-11.4). The fraction of the target population that has actually received this schedule of vaccinations reached 28.1 percent in 2012, 32.7 percent in 2013, and 34.4 percent in 2014, the last year for which data are available (HealthyPeople.gov 2017a). Vaccination rates were even lower for males between the ages of 13 and 15—6.9 percent in 2012, 13.5 percent in 2013, and 20.6 percent in 2014 (HealthyPeople.gov 2017b, IID-11.5). How does one account for these low rates of vaccination, especially in view of the vaccination rates for most other infectious diseases.

A number of scholarly studies have been conducted to answer this question, and it appears that a variety of answers is possible (for example, see Gilkey et al. 2015; Holman et al. 2014; White 2014). One such concern that was expressed even before the HPV vaccine was approved was that its availability would increase the risk of promiscuity in women. The argument was that if a woman knew that she was protected against sexual disease and, hence, cervical cancer, she would be more likely to engage in more and a greater variety of sexual experiences. For example, in 2005, Bridge Maher of the Family Research Council, a conservative Christian-based organization told a reporter from the *New Scientist* journal that "giving the HPV vaccine to young women could be potentially harmful, because they may see it as a license to engage in premarital sex" (MacKenzie 2005; also see Schwartz and Kempner 2015, 183–189).

That argument was largely laid to rest in a study reported in 2012. In that research, the sexual behaviors of a total of 1,398 girls, of whom 493 had received the HPV vaccine and 905 who had not, were studied. Results of the study indicated that there was no difference between the two groups on this criterion.

The authors concluded that "receipt of HPV vaccine by 11- to 12-year-old girls was not associated with clinical markers of increased sexual activity–related outcomes, such as sexually transmitted diseases or pregnancy" (Bednarczyk et al. 2012).

Another argument for avoiding the use of the HPV vaccine is that the vaccine itself has not been adequately been tested, is not safe, and is responsible for numerous injuries and deaths since its introduction in 2006. Radio talk host and founder of the Progressive Radio Network, Gary Null, for example, has taken such a position in his presentation, "HPV Vaccines: Unnecessary and Lethal." In this piece, Null argues that:

> Since Gardasil's launch in 2006 until November 2012, the HPV vaccine was linked to 121 deaths and over 27,485 medical injuries of young girls, some as young as 11 years old. At the end of last year, the number rose to over 30,000 serious injuries and over 150 deaths. Unfortunately, only a fraction of vaccine adverse events reported by pediatricians, physicians, medical clinics and hospitals, make their way into the VAERS [Vaccine Adverse Events Reporting System] database. Few parents even know such a reporting system exists. (Null n.d.)

Null then goes on to list a number of medical conditions that he claims can result from HPV vaccinations: acute juvenile rheumatoid arthritis, autoimmune disorders, encephalopathy, and fatal infections of the brain.

Similar accusations can be found on a number of sources on the Internet. One reviewer, for example, has announced that the "once held theory" that the HPV vaccine was safe had now "officially been proved false" (Jaxen 2016). The reviewer cites a number of individual and group statements that dispute claims of safety, argue that FDA approval of the vaccine was based on fraud, and warn that "young women are dying and losing their ability to have children" as a result of exposure to the vaccine (Jaxen 2016, with about two dozen links to reports of individual specific cases of supposed medical harm resulting from the vaccine).

Claims such as these have been contested by a number of agencies who have in the past promoted the use of the vaccine. The CDC, for example, has acknowledged that a number of side effects may be associated with an HPV vaccination, as is the case with any type of vaccination. But these are generally low-level effects such as pain, redness, or swelling in the arm where the shot was given; fever; headache or feeling tired; nausea; and muscle or joint pain (CDC 2016f). With regard to claims of more serious health effects and deaths as a result of receiving the vaccine, the CDC points out that nearly 90 million doses of the vaccine were given between June 2006 and March 2016. During that time, 35,624 reports of adverse effects were reported to Vaccine Adverse Events Reporting System, the vast majority of which involved the relatively minor effects noted above. About 7 percent of all adverse results were classified as "serious," prompting more detailed study and analysis by the CDC.

Such research is very difficult because one cannot always associate a particular adverse effect with a vaccination. That is, a person may become ill for some reason other than the HPV vaccine after the vaccination has occurred. As a result of its investigations, however, the CDC concluded that there was insufficient evidence to associate use of the vaccine with any of the adverse effects most commonly mentioned by critics, including ovarian failure, infertility, Guillain-Barré syndrome (an autoimmune disorder), or postural orthostatic tachycardia syndrome (light-headedness, fainting, and rapid heartbeat). The CDC also concluded that studies of mortalities claimed to result from an HPV vaccination could not be confirmed and that "there is no diagnosis that would suggest Gardasil caused the death" in any of the cases for which that result was claimed (CDC 2017a).

Many individuals and some organizations also oppose the use, especially mandates, of HPV vaccines. They argue that, yes, thousands of women may die every year as a result of cervical cancer, but that statistic hardly represents a compelling reason for using an inadequately tested, unsafe, probably ineffective vaccine. After all, cervical cancer rates have been dropping for years and the introduction of such a potentially harmful health product such as the HPV vaccine is hardly justified. Critics in a number of countries in addition to the United States have been making that argument since 2006, and are continuing to do so today (see, for example, Auckland Women's Health Council 2008 [New Zealand]; Irish Times 2010 [Ireland]; Judicial Watch 2008; Spring 2013 [Canada]).

The debate over the use of the HPV vaccine is not limited to the United States. In Japan, for example, the government withdrew its recommendation for HPV vaccination in 2013 because of reports of serious adverse effects among girls who had been given the vaccine. As a consequence, vaccination rate in the country dropped from about 70 percent to about 1 percent (Nelson 2016). Opposition to the vaccine was strong in other nations also. In 2015, health officials in Denmark discontinued use of Gardasil because of reports of adverse health effects and replaced the vaccine with Cervarix in its HPV vaccination program (Nsnbc International 2015; Danish Health Authority 2016). Five years earlier the Indian government had also discontinued a demonstration project for the HPV vaccine. Strong opposition from a number of advocacy groups was generally blamed for that decision (Larson, Brocard, and Garnett 2010). Controversy over the use of the vaccine also continues in a number of other countries, including Colombia, Ireland, France, Scotland, South Africa, and Spain (Shilhavey 2017).

Despite substantial expressions of concern about the safety and efficacy of the HPV vaccine, virtually all professional organizations concerned with public health issues, STIs, cervical cancer, and related issues continue to recommend the use of the vaccine for young boys and girls and most adolescents. One modification that was announced in October 2016 was the use of a two-dose vaccine for all 11- and 12-year-olds, rather than the previous recommendation of three doses (American Academy of Family Physicians 2017; American Cancer Society 2016; CDC 2016a; Jenco 2016; National Cancer Institute 2016).

Still other objections have been raised about the use of HPV vaccines, especially the questions of freedom of choice and cost of the procedure. The argument is that the use of the HPV vaccine, especially mandates for its use, violates a parent's rights to make decisions as to the type of health and medical care, if any, that a child should receive. After all, parents are ultimately responsible for their children, and in questions as to their physical, mental, and emotional care, ultimate decisions should be left to them. This argument is to some extent a part of the general opposition to all or most types of vaccinations now required of nearly all school children. The range of arguments against vaccination is now quite extensive, including the following:

- Vaccines are often not needed for diseases that are now largely under control.
- Vaccines themselves often cause serious adverse effects, which may include death.
- Vaccines may include "inactive" ingredients that add nothing to their preventive potential, but that may cause health issues in and of themselves.
- Requiring a child to be vaccinated may interfere with a person's religious beliefs.
- Governmental bodies are overstepping their limits of action by requiring students to be vaccinated.
- Vaccines are synthetic substances that may not be as effective as natural products that have been used to prevent and treat diseases (ProCon.org 2017).

Proponents of required vaccination reject these views and argue that all generally available vaccines are safe and efficacious. As

Dr. Martin Myers, executive director of the National Network for Immunization Information, has said, "there is in fact no credible 'controversy' about the safety or effectiveness of the currently US licensed childhood vaccines. Rather, some uninformed and misinformed individuals have articulated scientifically unsubstantiated claims about vaccines" (Newton 2013, 114–115). Indeed, some leaders of the public health profession have decided that it may be best simply to ignore the arguments of the anti-vaccinationists and to proceed with established programs of mandatory vaccination in all settings in which they are appropriate.

In spite of this type of expert opinion about vaccinations, opponents of required HPV vaccinations continue to voice their objections to the practice. For example, the decision of the Rhode Island Department of Health to institute an HPV vaccination requirement in all public schools in the state produced a renewed campaign by opponents of the mandate (Freyer 2015; Rhode Island Center for Freedom and Prosperity 2015; also see Vermont Coalition for Vaccine Choice 2017).

HIV: An Epidemic under Control?

Many people alive in 2017 have little memory of the rise of HIV infections in the United States. The disease appeared on the scene in 1981, when 270 cases of the disease were reported in the United States. By the following year, that number had risen to 452 and then to 3,064 in 1983 and 15,948 in 1984. Overall, between 1981 and 1987, 50,280 individuals had been diagnosed with the disease, of whom 47,993 (95.5%) had died. Over the next five-year period, the number of cases had risen by 202,520, of whom 181,212 (89.5%) had died of the disease. (Estimates of the number of HIV/AIDS cases is complicated by the fact that the CDC has changed the definition of an "HIV/AIDS case" a number of times over the past three decades. For example, the latest CDC report resulted in a finding that such cases had dropped by 18 percent between 2008 and 2014, considerably more than had previously been listed. See CDC 2017c.)

Better education and the development of a successful retroviral therapy rather dramatically affected these numbers. While another 264,405 cases of HIV were diagnosed between 1996 and 2000, the death rate had dropped to 22.6 percent, or 59,807 individuals. The number of new HIV infections has gradually leveled off at about 40,000 per year (CDC 2013, Table 1a; 2016d, Table 1a; *MMWR* 2001, Table 1).

In terms of absolute numbers, then, HIV might be thought of as a disease relatively under control. But STI specialists are disappointed in current trends of new cases. In the first place, an estimated 1.2 million people in the United States are living with the infection, of whom perhaps one in eight are not even aware of their HIV status. Successful treatment of the disease depends very much on early diagnosis and treatment of the infection. One major objective of current STI educational programs, then, is to encourage everyone who may be risk for the disease to have regular checkups to monitor their health status.

Another concern is that the rate of infection for HIV for certain groups at greatest risk has gradually been inching its way up over the past decade. This trend is especially true for Latino MSM, among whom the rate of infection has increased by 24 percent from 2008 to 2014; among Asian American MSM, by 101 percent during that period; among the American Indian/Alaska Native MSM population by 63 percent; among black and Latino men between the ages of 13 and 24, who experienced an increase in rate of HIV by 87 percent for both groups; and among white MSM between the ages of 13 and 24, where the increase was 56 percent (CDC Fact Sheet 2016).

Whatever success in dealing with the HIV epidemic has occurred depends to a large extent on a number of drugs that have been developed to combat the virus that causes the disease. Currently the FDA has approved more than 40 drugs for the treatment of HIV infection, drugs that are used in various combinations with each other. Maintaining a strict schedule in the use of these drugs is crucial to their effectiveness. But when used properly, they generally allow a person who is HIV positive to live a relatively normal and long life (AIDSinfo 2017; AIDS.gov 2015).

One of the most successful programs for the prevention of HIV/AIDS has been the so-called PrEP (for pre-exposure prophylaxis) agenda. This program is designed for individuals who have not yet been diagnosed with the disease, but who are considered to be a "high risk" for infection. "High risk" is defined by the CDC as:

- Anyone who is in an ongoing sexual relationship with an HIV-infected partner.
- A gay or bisexual man who has had sex without a condom or has been diagnosed with an STI within the past six months, and is not in a mutually monogamous relationship with a partner who recently tested HIV negative.
- A heterosexual man or woman who does not always use condoms when having sex with partners known to be at risk for HIV (for example, injecting drug users or bisexual male partners of unknown HIV status), and is not in a mutually monogamous relationship with a partner who recently tested HIV negative.
- Anyone who has, within the past six months, injected illicit drugs and shared equipment or been in a treatment program for injection drug use (CDC 2014).

The PrEP program calls for a person to take one pill every day of the drug Truvada˚, which consists of two antiviral medications, tenofovir and emtricitabine. Research has shown that people who adhere to this regimen very conscientiously may reduce their risk of contracting HIV by as much as 92 percent, although that level of protection drops significantly for anyone who does not stay on schedule (Scott and Klausner 2016).

One of the concerns first expressed about the PrEP program was that it might lead to more risky sexual behavior by the individuals in the at-risk population. That is, the question was raised as to whether a person who was on the regimen might feel safe enough to engage in risky sexual behavior and, therefore, actually *increase* his or her participation in such behavior. Enough studies have now been done to confirm that this concern is unwarranted: Individuals taking Truvada° turn out not to engage in risky behavior any more often than those who are not on the regimen (Marcus et al. 2013).

Another interesting question that has come up about the PrEP program goes back to the early days of the AIDS crisis: what connection, if any, is there between HIV infections and other types of STIs? There is some logic to believing that such an association may exist and that having an STI may increase the risk of a person's being infected by HIV. In the first place, some people argued, STIs and AIDS both occur as the result of well-known sexual behaviors. People who have many sexual partners and/or take no precautions in the sexual activities (such as not wearing a condom) are more likely to contract both STIs and AIDS. A biological reason to believe in the hypothesis also exists. Many forms of STIs are characterized by lesions in the skin, providing an easy mechanism by which the AIDS virus can be transmitted during sexual activities. Indeed, a number of studies have confirmed that this relationship does exist (see, for example, Galvin and Cohen 2004).

Recent research has confirmed the association of STIs with HIV infections. As an example, one study showed that individuals with two prior cases of rectal gonorrhea or chlamydia were eight times more likely to develop an HIV infection than were members of a control group (Bernstein et al. 2010). This type of finding appears to explain rising rates of syphilis and gonorrhea among MSM discussed earlier in this chapter. They further emphasize the necessity of improving the understanding of at-risk populations of the methods and risks of STI/HIV transmissions (Scott and Klausner 2016).

An obvious step in the battle against HIV/AIDS—a vaccine against the virus—was initiated shortly after the virus was discovered in 1983. (For a good overview of efforts to develop an HIV/AIDS vaccine, see Esparza 2013.) In 1984, Secretary of Health and Human Services, Margaret Heckler, announced that the virus responsible for AIDS had been discovered. In her press conference announcing the discovery, Heckler was also asked about the possibility of a vaccine for the disease. She said that she had been advised that a vaccine could be developed "within two years" (Frontline 2006). That prediction surprised most scientists and journalists because development of a new vaccine takes a decade or more. As it turns out, the skeptics were correct on this point. As of late 2017, more than 30 years had passed without success in developing such a vaccine. A number of candidates had been suggested and tested, but none had met the standards of (1) safety to people who are vaccinated and (2) efficacy in preventing the disease.

From the outset, most experts recognized that development of an AIDS vaccine would have to be a multi-institutional project. No one laboratory had the resources of experiences to attack this problem. As early as 1988, then, the U.S. National Institutes of Health created the AIDS Vaccine Evaluation Group designed to provide a way of testing vaccines that had been developed. Eight years later, the group announced that it had already reviewed "16 experimental AIDS vaccines, 10 adjuvants (a substance that enhances the immune responses stimulated by a vaccine), and a variety of delivery vehicles and routes, dosages and schedules of immunization" (National Institutes of Health 2006).

In 1996, Anthony Fauci, director of the National Institute of Allergy and Infectious Diseases, listed the reasons that development of an AIDS vaccine was such a challenge. He cited the following factors:

- Classic vaccines mimic natural immunity against reinfection generally seen in individuals recovered from infection; there are no recovered AIDS patients.

- Most vaccines protect against disease, not against infection; HIV infection may remain latent for long periods before causing AIDS.

- Most vaccines provide protection for years against viruses that change very little over time; HIV-1 mutates at a rapid rate and efficiently selects mutant forms that evade immunity.

- Most effective vaccines are whole-killed or live-attenuated organisms killed; HIV-1 does not retain antigenicity and the use of a live retrovirus vaccine raises safety issues.

- Most vaccines protect against infections that are infrequently encountered; HIV may be encountered daily by individuals at high risk.

- Most vaccines protect against infections through mucosal surfaces of the respiratory or gastrointestinal tract; the great majority of HIV infection is through the genital tract.

- Most vaccines are tested for safety and efficacy in an animal model before trials with human volunteers; there is no suitable animal model for HIV/AIDS at the present (adapted from Fauci 1996, as cited in Kindt, Goldsby, and Osborne 2007, 519).

Frustrations over the failure to develop an HIV/AIDS vaccine appeared to have been salved in 2009 with reports that a vaccine known as RV144 was found to be moderately effective in preventing HIV infections and AIDS among a population of Thai individuals at risk for the disease. Researchers concluded that what they regarded as "the first effective vaccine against HIV" (American Chemical Society 2012) "provided preliminary evidence that an HIV vaccine regimen has the potential to prevent infection." A potential problem, they noted, was that RV144 "did not have the power to address two intriguing considerations: vaccine efficacy may have decreased over the first year after vaccination, and vaccine efficacy may have been greater in persons at lower risk for infection" (Rerks-Ngarm et al. 2009; a report on this research is available from the sponsoring agency, the U.S. Military HIV Research Program 2017).

The two concerns expressed by authors of the so-called Thai study were troubling enough to call for further studies of the efficacy of RV144 in the human population (Sheets, Zhou, and Knezevic 2016, 84). As a consequence, new trials were scheduled to begin in South Africa in 2016 to obtain further information on the potential of RV144 as an HIV/AIDS vaccine (Boseley 2016; National Institutes of Health 2016a).

Vaccine Successes: Hepatitis

Hope for the discovery of vaccines for various STIs is based to some extent on the record of success of two such vaccines already available, the hepatitis A vaccine and the hepatitis B vaccine. The latter became commercially available in the United States in 1982, while the former was first released for use in 1995. As shown in Table 2.6, as each vaccine became more widely available, its success in reducing the incidence of the two diseases became readily apparent. The peak rate of hepatitis B occurred in 1985 (11.5 cases per 100,000), shortly after release of the vaccine, and then began to fall off to its current rate of 0.9 cases per 100,000. The same pattern has been observed for hepatitis A, for which the infection rate was 14.4 cases per 100,000 in 1989 before beginning to fall after release of the vaccine to its current rate of 0.4 cases per 100,000.

The contrast between the types of hepatitis against which there are and are not vaccines is illustrated by comparison with infection rates for hepatitis C (formerly known as not-A-not-B hepatitis). Hepatitis C appeared, like hepatitis A and hepatitis B, to be coming under control after 1992, when rates were 2.4 per 100,000. But then, after those rates had bottomed out at around 0.3 per 100,000 in the early 2000s, they began to rise again to their current rate of 0.7 per 100,000, a rate that has more than doubled in the five years between 2009 and 2014 (all data from annual surveillance surveys by the CDC 2016h).

Table 2.6   Incidence and Rate of Hepatitis A, B, and C, 1966–2014

Year	Hepatitis A Number	Hepatitis A Rate[1]	Hepatitis B Number	Hepatitis B Rate[1]	Hepatitis C Number	Hepatitis C Rate[1]
1966	32,859	16.8	1,497	0.8	—[2]	—[2]
1967	38,909	19.7	2,458	1.3	—	—
1968	45,893	23.0	4,829	2.5	—	—
1969	48,416	24.0	5,909	3.0	—	—
1970	56,797	27.9	8,310	4.1	—	—
1971	59,606	28.9	9,556	4.7	—	—
1972	54,074	26.0	9,402	4.5	—	—
1973	50,749	24.2	8,451	4.0	—	—
1974	40,358	19.5	10,631	5.2	—	—
1975	35,855	16.8	13,121	6.3	—	—
1976	33,288	15.5	14,973	7.1	—	—
1977	31,153	14.4	16,831	7.8	—	—
1978	29,500	13.5	15,016	6.9	—	—
1979	30,407	13.8	15,452	7.0	—	—
1980	29,087	12.8	19,015	8.4	—	—
1981	25,802	11.3	21,152	9.2	—	—
1982	23,403	10.1	22,177	9.6	2,629[3]	1.1[3]
1983	21,532	9.2	24,318	10.4	3,470	1.5
1984	22,040	9.3	26,115	11.1	3,871	1.6
1985[4]	23,257	10.0	26,654	11.5	4,192	1.8
1986[4]	23,430	10.0	26,107	11.2	3,634	1.6
1987	25,280	10.4	25,916	10.7	2,999	1.2
1988	28,507	11.6	23,177	9.4	2,619	1.1
1989	35,821	14.4	23,419	9.4	2,529	1.0
1990	31,441	12.6	21,102	8.5	2,553	1.0
1991	24,378	9.7	18,003	7.1	3,582	1.4
1992	23,112	9.1	16,126	6.3	6,010	2.4
1993	24,238	9.4	13,361	5.2	4,786	1.9
1994	26,796	10.3	12,517	4.8	4,470	1.8
1995	31,582	12.0	10,805	4.1	4,576	1.7
1996	31,032	11.7	10,637	4.0	3,716	1.4

(continued)

Table 2.6 (Continued)

Year	Hepatitis A		Hepatitis B		Hepatitis C	
	Number	Rate[1]	Number	Rate[1]	Number	Rate[1]
1997	30,021	11.2	10,416	3.9	3,816	1.4
1998	23,229	8.6	10,258	3.8	3,518	1.3
1999	17,047	6.3	7,694	2.8	3,111	1.1
2000	13,397	4.8	8,036	2.9	3,197	1.1
2001	10,615	3.7	7,844	2.8	1,640[5]	0.7[5]
2002	8,795	3.1	8,064	2.8	1,223[6]	0.5[6]
2003	7,653	2.6	7,526	2.6	891[6]	0.3[6]
2004	5,683	1.9	6,212	2.1	758	0.3
2005	4,488	1.5	5,494	1.8	694	0.2
2006	3,579	1.2	4,713[7]	1.6[7]	802	0.3
2007[8]	2,979	1.0	4,519	1.5	849	0.3
2008	2,585	0.9	4,029	1.3	877	0.3
2009	1,987	0.6	3,371	1.1	781	0.3
2010	1,670	0.5	3,350	1.1	850	0.3
2011	1,398	0.4	2,903	0.9	1,232	0.4
2012	1,562	0.5	2,895	0.9	1,778	0.6
2013	1,781	0.6	3,050	1.0	2,138	0.7
2014	1,239	0.4	2,791	0.9	2,194	0.7

Source: Centers for Disease Control and Prevention. 206. "Statistics and Surveillance." https://www.cdc.gov/hepatitis/statistics/. Accessed on February 24, 2017.

[1] Per 100,000.

[2] Not a reportable disease until 1982.

[3] Date from 1982 through 1991 are unreliable.

Data unavailable for New York City;[4] New Jersey and Missouri;[5] Missouri;[6] Arizona;[7] District of Columbia.[8]

All forms of hepatitis may occur either as an acute or as a chronic condition. In the case of hepatitis B, infants and children are at considerable risk (more than 90% for the former and 25–50% for the latter), while such is not the case for adults (generally less than 10%). Hepatitis C presents a quite different picture, with anywhere between 75 and 85 percent of all acute cases eventually advancing to the chronic stage (WHO 2016a).

As its name suggests (*hepa* = "liver"; *-titis* = "inflammation") the liver is the primary organ of concern in all forms of hepatitis. The amount of damage done, however, varies considerably, from essentially none in the case of hepatitis A to moderate (about a quarter of all chronic cases) for hepatitis B and severe (as many as three quarters of all chronic cases) for hepatitis C. The long-term effects of any type of hepatitis, insofar as it poses a threat to one's health, includes cirrhosis, cancer of the liver, liver failure, and chronic liver disease.

One can perhaps summarize the story of hepatitis at the present time as follows. While no infectious disease can ever be thought of as harmless, the health concerns posed by hepatitis A and hepatitis B are relatively modest. Especially in their acute stages, they pose little bodily harm and seldom advance to more serious chronic phases. The story line for hepatitis C is very different. The rates for this form of the infection have continued to rise, not only worldwide, but also in the United States. A study reported in 2016, for example, found that the incidence of hepatitis C in the 10-year period between 2003 and 2013 nearly doubled, from 11,051 to 19,368. At that point the number of deaths from the disease exceeded the total number of deaths from 60 other nationally notifiable infectious conditions (ONNICs), which amounted to 17,915. Additionally, the trend of the total number of ONNICs in the United States has been shifting downward for many years, while that for hepatitis C has been going in the other direction (Ly et al. 2016).

How does one explain this trend? A number of factors are involved. In the first place, a large fraction of individuals infected with HAC are unaware of the condition. They have no symptoms and, therefore, no reason to expect that they have the virus. This fact means that many individuals who go on to the chronic stage of hepatitis C have not and will not obtain antiviral counseling and therapy that is available, but about which they are uninterested until the disease has reached an advanced state. In the majority of cases, hepatitis C is not even listed on death certificates of those who have died as a result of the disease (Mahajan et al. 2014).

Another reason for the trend may be that the vast majority of the world population and those in the United States do not yet understand the course of a hepatitis C infection. Estimates place at 3.5 million the number of individuals infected with hepatitis C in the United States, of whom only about half are aware of their status (CDC 2016e). The disease may be dormant in a person for many decades before it becomes active and the individual becomes symptomatic. At that point, the person, and even his or her health care provider, may not be aware that current health problems can be traced back many years to an earlier infection. Yet a third factor may be the increase in incidence of injection drug use in the United States and elsewhere. A number of studies in the United States have shown that the proportion of individuals infected with hepatitis C are white adults under the age of 30 with a previous history of injection drug use (Page et al. 2013).

Treatments for hepatitis C have been available for some time. Until quite recently, the drugs of choice were injectable interferon and one of a group of oral drugs, including Harvoni, Solvadi, Epclusa, Zepatier, Boceprevir, and Telaprevir. The last two of these medications have been discontinued, however, because of the long treatment they require (up to six months) and severe side effects. That leaves eight oral medications and two injectable drugs available for use against hepatitis C. All are reasonably, if not universally, successful in treating the infection. One of the most serious problems with the use of these medications, however, is their cost. Harvoni, for example, is sometimes called "the most expensive drug in America," with the cost of a 30-day supply listed at $87,800. The next three most expensive drugs are also hepatitis C medications: Solvadi, at $73,800 for a three-month supply; Epclusa, $73,300; and Zepatier, $52,600 (GoodRx 2017; exact prices vary depending on the source of the drug and other factors).

In light of the high cost of such drugs, prevention efforts against hepatitis C are of special importance. Such efforts focus, as one might expect, on educational programs in which individuals at risk, as well as the general public, are informed about the nature of the disease, its possible outcomes, and ways in which it can be prevented. In the case of this type of hepatitis, however, one other approach to prevention has also been developed: needle (or syringe) exchange programs. A needle exchange program targets individuals who inject drugs intravenously (IV users) and who are, therefore, at high risk for infection with HCV. According to one source, IV drug users now represent the largest group on individuals at risk for HCV infection. A variety of studies have found that anywhere from 50 to 100 percent of IV drugs users who were studied eventually developed the disease (Dartmouth Medical School 2017).

In a needle exchange program, an IV drug user brings one or more needles or syringes that he or she has used for drug injection to an exchange site. At that site, a governmental or private agency accepts those needles, destroys them, and provides the user with clean needles. The exchange process may also involve other forms of drug paraphernalia, such as cookers and filters (Ontario Harm Reduction Distribution Program 2017).

Needle exchange programs began in Amsterdam in 1984 when a major pharmacy in the city stopped selling needles and syringes to known IV drug users. The federal government decided to institute an exchange program as a way of avoiding the most serious issues that IV drug users face. By this point in time, it was already apparent that one such problem was AIDS. Research studies had already made it clear that sharing of needles by drug users was a major method by which the new disease was transmitted. The Dutch concept soon spread throughout a number of other developed nations, and by 2008, 77 countries worldwide had adopted such a program. By that time, the goal of needle exchange programs was to reduce not only the spread of HIV/AIDS, but also the transmission of hepatitis C (Cook and Kanaef 2008, Table A.3. page 15).

The United States had, by that time, adopted needle exchange programs in many parts of the country. That step had not occurred easily, however, as opposition to such programs was very strong for many years following the Amsterdam experiment. The most common argument made by opponents was that by providing free, clean needles to IV drug users, the government was only encouraging further drug use. That theme remains influential today; as of June 2014, 17 states have laws explicitly banning needle exchange programs within their borders. In 11 other states and the District of Columbia, only one such program exists within the state or district (North American Syringe Exchange Network 2017; for an excellent review of the history of needle exchange programs in the United States up to 2007, see Bassler 2007).

The question as to the effectiveness of needle exchange programs has been the subject of many research endeavors, with apparently no clear-cut answers. As far back as the early 1990s, researchers began to measure the efficacy of needle exchange programs in reducing the incidence and prevalence of both HIV and hepatitis C infections (Substance Abuse and Mental Health Services Administration n.d.). In sum, those studies appeared to show that such programs do have significant effects on the rate of infection for both diseases. More recent research has produced essentially the same results (Hagan, Pouget, and Des Jarlais 2011). One of the most recent meta-analyses of 15 studies of the efficacy of needle exchange programs in reducing HIV and HCV infection, for example, concluded that the overall results of these studies "support NSP as a structural-level intervention to reduce population-level infection and implementation of NSP for prevention and treatment of HIV and HCV infection" (Abdul-Quader et al. 2013).

In recognition of these results, the U.S. Congress in 2016 adopted legislation that would support the expansion of these programs. The bill, the Consolidated Appropriations Act of 2016, does not permit the use of federal funds to purchase sterile needles. However, it does allow cities and states to apply for grants to support other aspects of such programs (Department of Health and Human Services 2016b).

Another area of progress in dealing with hepatitis C involves the development of a vaccine for the disease. Given the success of HAV and HBV vaccines, it would seem only natural for researchers to be working on a vaccine for HCV also. And, in fact, vaccine research began very soon after the discovery of the HCV. But progress has been slow, and, as of 2017, no HCV vaccine is yet available. The failure to produce a vaccine is the consequence of a number of factors that often arise in the development of a vaccine: HCV evolves and changes more rapidly than do the HAV and HBV; there are relatively few animals that can be used in experiments on a trial vaccine; it is difficult to recruit people to take part in vaccine trials; and, as noted above, HCV does not produce antigens that can clearly be used as "markers" that a vaccine can attack.

But there are signs of hope. In 2015, for example, a team of researchers from the United States and Denmark reported on the existence of HCV-like viruses in a number of animals—including bats, rodents, monkeys, and horses—that might eventually be used as model subjects for a human vaccine. That step would help solve at least one of the challenges noted above (Scheel et al. 2015). In addition, research on humans seems to be moving forward, albeit very slowly. There are currently fewer than a half dozen vaccine candidates undergoing clinical trials. None of these vaccines have yet gone past stage III of clinical tests (Abdelwahab and Said 2016). Clinical testing of a new drug involves four stages, ranging from testing for safety in a small number of volunteers to testing for efficacy in a large group of volunteers (for more on this topic, see U.S. Food and Drug Administration 2015; for a description of one HCV vaccine trial, see National Institutes of Health 2016b).

The Silent Epidemic: Herpes

The term *herpes* is used to describe two closely related STIs caused by a pair of viruses, known as herpes simplex viruses

(HSV). Herpes simplex virus 1 (HSV-1) is responsible for infections around the mouth, such as cold sores and fever blisters. It is transmitted by mouth-to-mouth contact, as occurs when two people kiss. Herpes simplex virus 2 (HSV-2) is the main cause of sores in the genital region, such as genital warts. It is transmitted primarily by sexual contact with an infected person (Herpes.com 2013). At one time, experts thought that the two forms of HSV stayed essentially in their "preferred" location: HSV-1 in mouth and HSV-2 in genitals. They now accept the fact that, although that characterization is largely correct, either virus can survive in either location. That means that a person with HSV-1 can transmit the virus to someone during oral sex, and vice versa (WebMD 2017).

Herpes is probably the most common STI in the United States and around the world. Current data suggest that as many as 90 percent of all Americans have been exposed to HSV-1 at some time in their lives, and between 50 and 80 percent have developed an active infection. One recent study has estimated that 3.709 billion people worldwide have contracted HSV-1, with the greatest exposure in Africa, Southeast Asia, and the Western Pacific region (Looker et al. 2015a,b). These numbers do not suggest any major public health problem, however, as most people are asymptomatic for the disease. They may develop a cold sore or fever blister from time to time, but the virus then "goes into hiding" (usually in sensory neurons in the body), and the symptoms disappear. However, the virus may reappear again at any time in the future, but without any serious or long-term health consequences (Grinde 2013).

A companion to the global study of HSV-1 was a similar study of the incidence and prevalence of HSV-2 worldwide. Authors of that study estimated that 417 million individuals worldwide are have been infected by the virus, again with the largest numbers in Africa, Southeast Asia, and the Western Pacific. They estimated that 19.2 million are infected annually. In the United States, the CDC estimates that 299,000 people were infected with HSV-2 in 2014, the most recent year for which data are available (CDC 2015b; estimates of the incidence and prevalence of both forms of herpes are inherently variable because neither disease is a reportable disease in the United States or elsewhere, so other means are used to develop such estimates. In the reference cited here, estimates come from visits to physicians' offices presenting with an HSV infection). Unlike most other STIs, no trend in incidence has been observed for HSV-2 infections over the past few decades (CDC 2017b; see Table 2.7).

Table 2.7   Incidence of Genital HSV-2 Infections in the United States, 1966–2014

Year	Number of Cases
1966	19,000
1967	15,000
1968	16,000
1969	15,000
1970	17,000
1971	49,000
1972	26,000
1973	51,000
1974	75,000
1975	36,000
1976	57,000
1977	116,000
1978	76,000
1979	83,000
1980	57,000
1981	133,000
1982	134,000
1983	106,000
1984	157,000
1985	124,000
1986	136,000

(continued)

Table 2.7   (Continued)

Year	Number of Cases
1987	102,000
1988	163,000
1989	148,000
1990	172,000
1991	235,000
1992	139,000
1993	172,000
1994	142,000
1995	160,000
1996	208,000
1997	176,000
1998	188,000
1999	224,000
2000	179,000
2001	157,000
2002	216,000
2003	203,000
2004	269,000
2005	266,000
2006	371,000
2007	317,000
2008	292,000
2009	306,000
2010	232,000
2011	227,000
2012	228,000
2013	306,000
2014	299,000

Source: Centers for Disease Control and Prevention. 2015. "Selected STDs and Complications—Initial Visits to Physicians' Offices, National Disease and Therapeutic Index, United States, 1966-2014." https://www.cdc.gov/std/stats15/tables/44.htm. Accessed on March 3, 2017.

The search for an HSV vaccine dates back almost a century. Shortly after the discovery of the virus that causes herpes, research began to look for a mechanism by which the disease could be avoided. One of the earliest of these efforts involved the use of a smallpox vaccine against herpes. It was unsuccessful, and the search has continued, without success, to the present day (Scott 1986). Some attempts, of course, have been more successful than others. One such candidate was greeted with optimism in the early 2010s when early studies showed that it was effective in protecting against herpes. However, those hopes were dashed in 2012 with reports of a very large study of 6,874 subjects in which the vaccine protected women no more effectively than did a placebo. (The results puzzled researchers since the candidate vaccine did protect subjects against HSV-1; Belshe 2012.) One of the most recent agents being tested is called GEN-003. It is currently in stage 2 clinical trials, with its parent company having announced successful completion of stage 1 and early stage 2 trials (Genocea Biosciences 2017; also see Bloom 2016).

Emerging Sexually Transmitted Diseases

Although progress against some traditional STIs has been encouraging to researchers, new threats have also begun to appear on the horizon. STIs about which we have known for some time, but not been regarded as serious health threats, have begun to assert themselves in a variety of settings. One such disease is lymphogranuloma venereum (LGV). The condition was first described in 1833 by Irish physician William Wallace (although English physician John Hunter may have provided an even earlier description, in 1786; Galbraith, Graham-Stewart, and Nicol 1957).

LGV is caused by variants of *C. trachomatis*, and is similar in its presentation to chancroid, HSV-2, and syphilis. It occurs among both women and men. The infection is endemic in many parts of the developing world, but relatively uncommon in developed nations. Reliable data on the disease in the United States are unavailable because the disease was removed from the CDC list of reportable conditions in 1995. In the preceding years, the incidence of the disease was reported as ranging from 185 in 1988 to a high of 471 in 1991 (*MMWR* 1996).

As with syphilis, three stages of LGV can be observed. In the first stage, small, painless papulae or pistules form in the genital regions that resolve without treatment after a few weeks. An infected person may very well not know that he or she has been infected. The second stage is characterized by swollen and painful lymph nodes, complicated by liver inflammation, pulmonary distress, cardiac disorders, and infections of the eye. After a period of latency, a third stage develops that is characterized primarily by proctocolitiis, an inflammation of the rectum and colon that is painful and accompanied by bloody discharges (Arsove 2016).

LGV belongs in the category of "emerging STIs" because of a number of outbreaks of the disease reported since 2003 in Australia, Europe, and North America. The first of these outbreaks occurred in Rotterdam in 2003, when a number of cases were reported from STI clinics. Prior to the outbreak, about five cases of LGV were seen in the country each year. In 2003, the number climbed to 13 (later adjusted to 65 cases for 2002/2003), followed by a further increase to 76 cases in 2004 (Koper et al. 2013; Van der Laar et al. 2006). Before long, the epidemic had spread to a number of other countries around the world, including the United States, the United Kingdom, Australia, and almost every Western European nation (Stoner and Cohen 2015). In every country, the raw number of cases was hardly overwhelming (usually in the few dozens or low hundreds), but the sudden reappearance and spread of the disease were of concern to specialists. The United Kingdom appears to have recorded the largest number of LGV cases since the 2004 outbreak, with a total of 2,138 cases having been reported between April 2003 and June 2012 (Hughes et al. 2013).

Perhaps the most remarkable finding about the epidemic was that the vast majority of individuals diagnosed with the disease were MSM. Many infected individuals reported having unprotected sex with their partners and were found to have coexisting STIs, such as gonorrhea or syphilis. These findings have prompted experts in the field to intensify education about LGV and the conditions under which it may occur with individuals at risk for the disease (Stoner and Cohen 2015).

A second emerging STD is an infection by the *Mycoplasma genitalium* bacterium. The microorganism was first identified in 1981, at which time it was found to be associated with non-gonococcal urethritis (NGU), a type of urethritis that is not caused by *N. gonorrhoeae*, the most common cause of NGU. *M. genitalium* is now thought to be responsible for about 20 percent of all NGU cases, 20–25 percent of all nonchlamydial NGU cases, and approximately 30 percent of all cases of persistent or recurrent urethritis (Taylor-Robinson and Jensen 2011). It is presently not known whether the disease has long-term, more serious consequences, such as infertility. The effect of *M. genitalium* on women is less clear at this point, although it appears to be implicated in about a fifth of all cases of cervicitis. It may also be associated with urethritis and PID (CDC 2015a).

As with LGV, precise numbers for the incidence and prevalence of *M. genitalium* in the United States are not available because the disease is not a legally reportable one. However, one detailed study has produced some apparently reliable data on the extent of the infection in this country. According to that study, about 16 percent of all females between the ages of 14 and 70 and 17 percent of all males tested positive for the organism. This number varied widely among different races and ethnicities, as well as from one age group to another. For example, the fraction of females by age varied from 2.9 percent among those in the 41–50 group to 30 percent for those in the 14–17 group. Among males, the lowest rate of infection was among the oldest age groups (0%) and highest among the youngest age groups (24% among the 21–30 age group; Getman et al. 2016, Table 1).

Conclusion

Some types of STIs are relatively innocuous. They may cause some physical discomfort or embarrassment, but they are generally not life threatening . . . not that *anyone* wants to have an STI! Other STIs are associated with far more serious health consequences, including death in the most extreme cases. So it is generally in almost everyone's interest to avoid contracting an STI.

Fortunately, that is an attainable goal. Individuals can take a number of precautions to avoid catching an STI, such as the following:

- Always use a latex condom during sexual activities.
- Know as much as possible about your prospective partner's sexual history.
- Limit the number of sexual partners one has; abstinence is the one certain way of avoiding an STI.
- Get vaccinated for diseases for which a vaccine is available.
- Avoid sexual activities that may lead to the physical conditions (such as tearing of tissue) that increase one's risk for an STI.
- Wash before one has sexual relationships.
- Get assistance if you are an intravenous drug user.

In general, the best way to avoid the problems outlined at the very beginning of Chapter 1 of this book is just to become better educated about the nature of STIs. Knowledge about such diseases is not a guarantee that one will never become infected; but it is one of the best first steps one can take to make sure that sexual experiences are safe and worry-free.

References

Abdelwahab, Kouka Saadeldin, and Zeinab Nabil Ahmed Said. 2016. "Status of Hepatitis C Virus Vaccination: Recent Update." *World Journal of Gastroenterology*, 22(2): 862–873. https://www.ncbi.nlm.nih.gov/pmc/articles/PMC4716084/. Accessed on March 1, 2017.

Abdul-Quader, A. S., et al. 2013. "Effectiveness of Structural-Level Needle/Syringe Programs to Reduce HCV and HIV Infection among People Who Inject Drugs: A Systematic Review." *AIDS and Behavior*, 17(9): 2878-2892.

AIDS.gov. 2015. "Overview of HIV Treatments." https://www.aids.gov/hiv-aids-basics/just-diagnosed-with-hiv-aids/treatment-options/overview-of-hiv-treatments/. Accessed on February 21, 2017.

AIDSinfo. 2017. "FDA-Approved HIV Medicines." https://aidsinfo.nih.gov/education-materials/fact-sheets/21/58/fda-approved-hiv-medicines. Accessed on February 21, 2017.

Allen, Vanessa G., et al. 2013. "*Neisseria Gonorrhoeae* Treatment Failure and Susceptibility to Cefixime in Toronto, Canada." *JAMA*, 309(2): 163–170.

American Academy of Family Physicians. 2017. "Human Papillomavirus Vaccine." http://www.aafp.org/patient-care/public-health/immunizations/disease-population/hpv.html. Accessed on February 21, 2017.

American Cancer Society. 2016. "American Cancer Society Recommendations for Human Papilloma Virus (HPV) Vaccine Use." https://www.cancer.org/cancer/cancer-causes/infectious-agents/hpv/acs-recommendations-for-hpv-vaccine-use.html. Accessed on February 21, 2017.

American Chemical Society. 2012. "Targeting Sugars in the Quest for a Vaccine against HIV—The Virus That Causes AIDS." https://www.acs.org/content/acs/en/pressroom/newsreleases/2012/august/

targeting-sugars-in-the-quest-for-a-vaccine-against-hiv-the-virus-that-causes-aids.html. Accessed on February 23, 2017.

Arsove, Pamela. 2016. "Lymphogranuloma Venereum." *Medscape.* http://emedicine.medscape.com/article/220869-overview#a4. Accessed on March 4, 2017.

Auckland Women's Health Council. 2008. "Gardasil." http://www.womenshealthcouncil.org.nz/Features/Hot+Topics/Gardasil.html. Accessed on February 20, 2017.

Bassler, Sara Elizabeth. 2007. "The History of Needle Exchange Programs in the United States." The University of Toledo Digital Repository. http://utdr.utoledo.edu/cgi/viewcontent.cgi?article=1274&context=graduate-projects. Accessed on February 26, 2017.

Bednarczyk, Robert A., et al. 2012. "Sexual Activity-related Outcomes after Human Papillomavirus Vaccination of 11- to 12-year-olds." *Pediatrics*, 130(5): 798–805. http://pediatrics.aappublications.org/content/130/5/798. Accessed on February 19, 2017.

Belshe, Robert B., et al. 2012. "Efficacy Results of a Trial of a Herpes Simplex Vaccine." *The New England Journal of Medicine*, 366(1): 34–43. http://www.nejm.org/doi/full/10.1056/NEJMoa1103151#t=article. Accessed on March 4, 2007.

Benedek, Thomas. n.d. "History of the Medical Treatment of Gonorrhea." *Infectious Disease and Microbial Agents.* http://www.antimicrobe.org/h04c.files/history/Gonorrhea.pdf. Accessed on February 10, 2017.

Bernstein, Kyle T., et al. 2010. "Rectal Gonorrhea and Chlamydia Reinfection Is Associated with Increased Risk of HIV Seroconversion." *Journal of Acquired Immune Deficiency Syndrome*, 53(4): 537–543. http://www.sfcityclinic.org/providers/rectalreinfection.pdf. Accessed on February 22, 2017.

Bibbins-Domingo, Kirsten, et al. 2016. "Screening for Syphilis Infection in Nonpregnant Adults and Adolescents: US Preventive Services Task Force Recommendation Statement." *JAMA*, 315(21): 2321–2327.

Bloom, Josh. 2016. "A Vaccine for Herpes Erupts in the News." American Council on Science and Health. http:// acsh.org/news/2016/03/10/vaccine-herpes-erupts-news-9932. Accessed on March 4, 2017.

Bolan, Gail. 2015. "Sexually Transmitted Disease Prevention." Centers for Disease Control and Prevention. http:// www.ncsddc.org/sites/default/files/docs/04_23_2015_ congressional_briefing_slides_bolan_final.pdf. Accessed on February 11, 2017.

Boseley, Sarah. 2016. "HIV Vaccine Test Hopes for Breakthrough in Combat against the Virus." *The Guardian*. https://www.theguardian.com/society/2016/nov/27/hiv-vaccine-test-hvtn702-virus-aids-southafrica. Accessed on February 23, 2017.

CDC Fact Sheet. 2016. "Trends in U.S. HIV Diagnoses, 2005-2014." https://www.cdc.gov/nchhstp/newsroom/ docs/factsheets/hiv-data-trends-fact-sheet-508.pdf. Accessed on February 21, 2017.

Centers for Disease Control and Prevention. 1999. "The National Plan to Eliminate Syphilis from the United States." Division of STD Prevention. https://www. cdc.gov/stopsyphilis/plan.pdf. Accessed on February 10, 2017.

Centers for Disease Control and Prevention. 2013. "Diagnoses of HIV Infection in the United States and Dependent Areas, 2012." https://www.cdc.gov/hiv/pdf/ statistics_2012_HIV_Surveillance_Report_vol_24.pdf. Accessed on February 21, 2017.

Centers for Disease Control and Prevention. 2014. "HIV PrEP Guidelines Press Release." https://www.cdc.gov/

nchhstp/newsroom/2014/PrEP-Guidelines-Press-Release.
html. Accessed on February 22, 2017.

Centers for Disease Control and Prevention. 2015a.
"Emerging Issues." https://www.cdc.gov/std/tg2015/
emerging.htm. Accessed on March 6, 2017.

Centers for Disease Control and Prevention. 2015b.
"Table 44. Selected STDs and Complications—Initial
Visits to Physicians' Offices, National Disease and
Therapeutic Index, United States, 1966-2014." https://
www.cdc.gov/std/stats15/tables/44.htm. Accessed on
March 3, 2017.

Centers for Disease Control and Prevention. 2016a.
"CDC Recommends Only Two HPV Shots for Young
Adolescents." https://www.cdc.gov/media/releases/2016/
p1020-hpv-shots.html. Accessed on February 21, 2017.

Centers for Disease Control and Prevention. 2016b. "Cervical
Cancer Statistics." https://www.cdc.gov/cancer/cervical/
statistics/. Accessed on February 17, 2017.

Centers for Disease Control and Prevention. 2016c.
"Chlamydia—CDC Fact Sheet (Detailed). https://www.
cdc.gov/std/chlamydia/stdfact-chlamydia-detailed.htm.
Accessed on February 15, 2017.

Centers for Disease Control and Prevention. 2016d.
"Diagnoses of HIV Infection in the United States and
Dependent Areas, 2015." https://www.cdc.gov/hiv/pdf/
library/reports/surveillance/cdc-hiv-surveillance-report-
2015-vol-27.pdf. Accessed on February 21, 2017.

Centers for Disease Control and Prevention. 2016e.
"Hepatitis C Kills More Americans Than Any Other
Infectious Disease." https://www.cdc.gov/media/
releases/2016/p0504-hepc-mortality.html. Accessed on
February 25, 2017.

Centers for Disease Control and Prevention. 2016f. "HPV
Vaccine Is Safe—(Gardasil)." https://www.cdc.gov/

vaccinesafety/pdf/data-summary-hpv-gardasil-vaccine-is-safe.pdf. Accessed on February 20, 2017.

Centers for Disease Control and Prevention. 2016g. "Overview of Budget Request," 1. https://www.cdc.gov/budget/documents/fy2017/fy-2017-cdc-budget-overview.pdf. Accessed on February 13, 2017.

Centers for Disease Control and Prevention. 2016h. "Statistics and Surveillance." https://www.cdc.gov/hepatitis/statistics/. Accessed on February 24, 2017.

Centers for Disease Control and Prevention. 2016i. "Table 1. Sexually Transmitted Diseases—Reported Cases and Rates of Reported Cases per 100,000 Population, United States, 1941–2015." https://www.cdc.gov/std/stats15/tables/1.htm. Accessed on February 15, 2017.

Centers for Disease Control and Prevention. 2016j. "2015 Sexually Transmitted Diseases Surveillance." https://www.cdc.gov/std/stats15/std-surveillance-2015-print.pdf. Accessed on February 10, 2017.

Centers for Disease Control and Prevention. 2017a. "Frequently Asked Questions about HPV Vaccine Safety." https://www.cdc.gov/vaccinesafety/vaccines/hpv/hpv-safety-faqs.html#A2. Accessed on February 20, 2017.

Centers for Disease Control and Prevention. 2017b. "Genital Herpes Screening." https://www.cdc.gov/std/herpes/screening.htm. Accessed on March 3, 2017.

Centers for Disease Control and Prevention. 2017c. "HIV Incidence: Estimated Annual Infections in the U.S., 2008-2014: Overall and by Transmission Route." https://www.cdc.gov/nchhstp/newsroom/docs/factsheets/hiv-incidence-fact-sheet_508.pdf. Accessed on March 2, 2017.

Centers for Disease Control and Prevention. 2017d. "Syphilis—CDC Fact Sheet (Detailed)." https://www.cdc.gov/std/syphilis/stdfact-syphilis-detailed.htm. Accessed on February 14, 2017.

Clement, Meredith E., and Charles B. Hicks. 2016. "Syphilis on the Rise: What Went Wrong?" *JAMA*, 315(21): 2281-2283. http://www.commed.vcu.edu/IntroPH/Communicable_Disease/2016/JAMA_STI_June.pdf. Accessed on February 12, 2017.

Committee on Infectious Diseases. 2007. "Prevention of Human Papillomavirus Infection: Provisional Recommendations for Immunization of Girls and Women with Quadrivalent Human Papillomavirus Vaccine." *Pediatrics*, 120(3): 666–668. http://pediatrics.aappublications.org/content/120/3/666. Accessed on February 18, 2017.

Committee on Infectious Diseases. 2012. "HPV Vaccine Recommendations." *Pediatrics*, 129(3): 602–605. http://pediatrics.aappublications.org/content/129/3/602. Accessed on February 18, 2017.

Cook, Catherine, and Natalya Kanaef. 2008. "The Global State of Harm Reduction 20008: Mapping the Response to Drug-Related HIV and Hepatitis C Epidemics." London: International Harm Reduction Association. https://www.hri.global/files/2014/10/20/GSHR-Report-2008.pdf. Accessed on February 26, 2017.

Crockett, Emily. 2017. "The GOP Obamacare Replacement Defunds Planned Parenthood and Restricts Abortion Coverage." *Vox*. http://www.vox.com/identities/2017/3/6/14836998/obamacare-repeal-replace-bill-defund-planned-parenthood. Accessed on March 7, 2017.

Danish Health Authority. 2016. "New HPV Vaccine in the Childhood Vaccination Programme." https://www.sst.dk/en/news/2016/new-hpv-vaccine-in-the-childhood-vaccination-programme. Accessed on February 20, 2017.

Dartmouth Medical School. 2017. "High Risk Groups—United States." http://www.epidemic.org/thefacts/

theepidemic/USRiskGroups/. Accessed on February 26, 2017.

Del Rio, Carlos, et al. 2012. "Update to CDC's Sexually Transmitted Diseases Treatment Guidelines, 2010: Oral Cephalosporins No Longer a Recommended Treatment for Gonococcal Infections." *Morbidity and Mortality Weekly*. Centers for Disease Control and Prevention. https://www. cdc.gov/MMWr/preview/mmwrhtml/mm6131a3.htm. Accessed on February 10, 2017.

Department of Health and Human Services. 2016a. Fiscal Year 2016: Centers for Disease Control and Prevention. Justification of Estimates for Appropriation Committees. https://www.cdc.gov/budget/documents/fy2016/fy-2016-cdc-congressional-justification.pdf. Accessed on February 11, 2017.

Department of Health and Human Services. 2016b. "Department of Health and Human Services Implementation Guidance to Support Certain Components of Syringe Services Programs, 2016." https:// www.aids.gov/pdf/hhs-ssp-guidance.pdf. Accessed on March 1, 2017.

Department of Health and Human Services. 2017. "CDC Budget Overview." https://www.hhs.gov/about/budget/ budget-in-brief/cdc/index.html#overview. Accessed on February 15, 2017.

Detels, Roger, et al. 2011. "The Incidence and Correlates of Symptomatic and Asymptomatic *Chlamydia trachomatis* and *Neisseria gonorrhoeae* Infections in Selected Populations in Five Countries." *Sexually Transmitted Diseases*, 38(6): 503–509. https://www.ncbi.nlm.nih.gov/ pmc/articles/PMC3408314/. Accessed on February 15, 2017.

Dukers-Muijrers, Nicole H. T. M., et al. 2012. "*Chlamydia trachomatis* Test-of-Cure Cannot Be Based on a Single

Highly Sensitive Laboratory Test Taken at Least 3 Weeks after Treatment." *PLoS ONE*, 7(3): e34108.

Entasis Therapeutics. 2017. "Pipeline." http://www.entasistx. com/pipeline/. Accessed on February 11, 2017.

Esparza, José. 2013. "A Brief History of the Global Effort to Develop a Preventive HIV Vaccine." *Vaccine*, 31(35): 3502–3518.

Executive Order RP65. 2007. http://www.lrl.state.tx.us/ scanned/govdocs/Rick%20Perry/2007/RP65.pdf. Accessed on February 18, 2017.

Farley, Robert. 2011. "More Bad Medicine in the Perry Vaccine Saga." FactCheck.org. http://www.factcheck. org/2011/09/more-bad-medicine-in-the-perry-vaccine-saga/. Accessed on February 18, 2017.

Fauci, Anthony S. 1996. "An HIV Vaccine: Breaking the Paradigms." *Proceedings of the Association of American Physicians*, 108(1): 6–13.

Freyer, Felice J. 2015. "Parents Protest R.I. Mandating HPV Vaccine for Teens." *The Boston Globe*. https://www. bostonglobe.com/metro/2015/09/07/rhode-island-mandate-for-hpv-vaccine-sparks-protests-and-interest-from-massachusetts-officials/ZKmTZNPVTVKibPgqsUAgYK/ story.html. Accessed on February 21, 2017.

Frontline. 2006. "Interview: Margaret Heckler." The Age of AIDS. http://www.pbs.org/wgbh/pages/frontline/ aids/interviews/heckler.html. Accessed on February 23, 2017.

Galbraith, H.-J. B., C. W. Graham-Stewart, and C. S. Nicol. 1957. "Lymphogranuloma Venereum." *British Medical Journal*, 2(5058): 1402–1405.

Galvin, Shannon R., and Myron S. Cohen. 2004. "The Role of Sexually Transmitted Diseases in HIV Transmission." *Nature Reviews Microbiology*, 2: 33–42. doi:10.1038/ nrmicro794.

Genocea Biosciences. 2017. "GEN-003." http://www. genocea.com/pipeline/gen003-for-genital-herpes/. Accessed on March 4, 2017.

Getman, Damon, et al. 2016. "*Mycoplasma genitalium* Prevalence, Coinfection, and Macrolide Antibiotic Resistance Frequency in a Multicenter Clinical Study Cohort in the United States." *Journal of Clinical Microbiology*, 54(9): 2278–2283. http://jcm.asm.org/ content/54/9/2278.full#T1. Accessed on March 7, 2017.

Gilkey, Melissa B., et al. 2015. "Physician Communication about Adolescent Vaccination: How Is Human Papillomavirus Vaccine Different?" *Preventive Medicine*, 77: 181–185.

Globocan. 2015. "Cervical Cancer: Estimated Incidence, Mortality and Prevalence Worldwide in 2012." http:// globocan.iarc.fr/old/FactSheets/cancers/cervix-new.asp. Accessed on February 18, 2017.

GoodR$_X$. 2017. "The GoodRx Top 10 (January 2017)." https://www.goodrx.com/drug-guide/expensive. Accessed on February 26, 2017.

Grinde, Bjørn. 2013. "Herpesviruses: Latency and Reactivation—Viral Strategies and Host Response." *Journal of Oral Microbiology*, 5(1): 1–9. https://www.ncbi.nlm.nih.gov/ pmc/articles/PMC3809354/. Accessed on March 3, 2017.

Hagan, Holly, Enrique R. Pouget, and Don C. Des Jarlais. 2011. "A Systematic Review and Meta-Analysis of Interventions to Prevent Hepatitis C Virus Infection in People Who Inject Drugs." *Journal of Infectious Diseases*, 204(1): 74–83. https://www.ncbi.nlm.nih.gov/pmc/ articles/PMC3105033/. Accessed on March 1, 2017.

Hahn, Andrew H., and David H. Spach. 2017. "Human Papillomavirus Infection." National STD Curriculum. http://www.std.uw.edu/go/pathogen-based/hpv/core-concept/all. Accessed on February 17, 2017.

HealthyPeople.gov. 2017a. "Female Adolescents Receiving 3+ Doses of HPV Vaccine by Age 13–15 years (Percent) by Total." HealthyPeople.gov. https://www.healthypeople. gov/2020/topics-objectives/topic/immunization-and-infectious-diseases/objectives. Accessed on February 19, 2017.

HealthyPeople.gov. 2017b. "Immunization and Infectious Diseases." https://www.healthypeople.gov/2020/topics-objectives/topic/immunization-and-infectious-diseases/ objectives. Accessed on February19, 2017.

Henry J. Kaiser Family Foundation. 2016. "U.S. Federal Funding for HIV/AIDS: Trends over Time." http://files. kff.org/attachment/Fact-Sheet-US-Federal-Funding-for-HIVAIDS-Trends-Over-Time. Accessed on February 15, 2017.

Herpes.com. 2013. "'Good' Virus/'Bad' Virus." http://www. herpes.com/hsv1-2.html. Accessed on March 3, 2017.

Holman, Dawn M., et al. 2014. "Barriers to Human Papillomavirus Vaccination among US Adolescents: A Systematic Review of the Literature." *JAMA Pediatrics*, 168(1): 76–82. https://www.ncbi.nlm.nih.gov/pmc/ articles/PMC4538997/. Accessed on February 19, 2017.

Hughes, G., et al. 2013. "Lymphogranuloma Venereum Diagnoses among Men Who Have Sex with Men in the U.K.: Interpreting a Cross-Sectional Study Using an Epidemic Phase-specific Framework." *Sexually Transmitted Infections*, 89(7): 542–547.

Immunization Action Coalition. 2016. "Give a Strong Recommendation for HPV Vaccine to Increase Uptake!" http://www.immunize.org/letter/recommend_hpv_ vaccination.pdf. Accessed on February 18, 2017.

Irish Times. 2010. "Is the Cervical Cancer Vaccine Good to Go?" *The Irish Times*. http://www.irishtimes.com/news/ health/is-the-cervical-cancer-vaccine-good-to-go-1.644917. Accessed on February 20, 2017.

Jaxen, Jeffrey. 2016. "American College of Pediatricians Latest to Warn of Gardasil HPV Vaccine Dangers." *Vaccine Impact*. https://vaccineimpact.com/2016/american-college-of-pediatricians-latest-to-warn-of-hpv-vaccine-dangers/. Accessed on February 20, 2017.

Jenco, Melissa. 2016. "ACIP Updates Recommendations on HPV, HepB, MenB Vaccines." American Academy of Pediatrics. http://www.aappublications.org/news/aapnewsmag/2016/10/20/ACIP102016.full.pdf. Accessed on February 21, 2017.

Jerse, Ann E., Margaret C. Bash, and Michael W. Russell. 2014. "Vaccines against Gonorrhea: Current Status and Future Challenges." *Vaccine*, 32(14): 1579-1587.

Judicial Watch. 2008. "Examining the FDA's HPV Vaccine Records." http://www.judicialwatch.org/wp-content/uploads/2014/02/JW-Report-FDA-HPV-Vaccine-Records.pdf. Accessed on February 20, 2017.

Kindt, Thomas J., Richard A. Goldsby, and Barbara A. Osborne. 2007. *Kuby Immunology*, 6th edition. New York: W. H. Freeman.

Kirkcaldy, R. D. 2013. "Treatment of Gonorrhoea in an Era of Emerging Cephalosporin Resistance and Results of a Randomised Trial of New Potential Treatment Options." *Sexually Transmitted Infections*, 89 (Suppl 1): A14.

Koper, N., et al. 2013. "Lymphogranuloma Venereum among Men Who Have Sex with Men in the Netherlands: Regional Differences in Testing Rates Lead to Underestimation of the Incidence, 2006-2012." *Eurosurveillance*, 18(34): 20561. http://www.eurosurveillance.org/images/dynamic/ee/v18n34/art20561.pdf. Accessed on March 5, 2017.

Kreisel, Kristen P., et al. 2017. "Prevalence of Pelvic Inflammatory Disease in Sexually Experienced Women of Reproductive Age—United States, 2013–2014." *Morbidity and Mortality Weekly Report*, 66(3): 80–83. https://www.

cdc.gov/mmwr/volumes/66/wr/mm6603a3.htm. Accessed on February 16, 2017.

Larson, Heidi J., Pauline Brocard, and Geoffrey Garnett. 2010. "The India HPV-vaccine Suspension." *Lancet*, 376(9741): 572–573. http://www.thelancet.com/pdfs/journals/lancet/PIIS0140-6736(10)60881-1.pdf. Accessed on February 20, 2017.

Liu, Yingru, Nejat K. Egilmez, and Michael W. Russell. 2013. "Enhancement of Adaptive Immunity to *Neisseria Gonorrhoeae* by Local Intravaginal Administration of Microencapsulated Interleukin 12." *The Journal of Infectious Diseases*, 208(11): 1821-1829.

Looker, Katharine, et al. 2015a. "Global Estimates of Prevalent and Incident Herpes Simplex Virus Type 1 Infections in 2012." *PLoS ONE*, 10(1): e0140765. http://journals.plos.org/plosone/article?id=10.1371/journal.pone.0140765. Accessed on March 3, 2017.

Looker, Katharine, et al. 2015b. "Global Estimates of Prevalent and Incident Herpes Simplex Virus Type 2 Infections in 2012." *PLoS ONE*, 10(1): e114989. http://journals.plos.org/plosone/article?id=10.1371/journal.pone.0114989. Accessed on March 3, 2017.

Ly, Kathleen, et al. 2016. "Rising Mortality Associated with Hepatitis C Virus in the United States, 2003–2013." *Clinical Infectious Diseases*, 62(10): 1287–1288. https://academic.oup.com/cid/article/62/10/1287/2462772/Rising-Mortality-Associated-With-Hepatitis-C-Virus. Accessed on February 25, 2017.

MacKenzie, Deborah. 2005. "Will Cancer Vaccine Get to All Women?" *New Scientist*. https://www.newscientist.com/article/mg18624954-500-will-cancer-vaccine-get-to-all-women/. Accessed on February 19, 2017.

Mahajan Reena, et al. 2014. "Mortality among Persons in Care with Hepatitis C Virus Infection: The Chronic

Hepatitis Cohort Study (CheCS), 2006–2010." *Clinical Infectious Diseases*, 58(8): 1055–1061.

Marcus, Julia L., et al. 2013. "No Evidence of Sexual Risk Compensation in the iPrEx Trial of Daily Oral HIV Preexposure Prophylaxis." *PLoS ONE*, 8(12): e81997. doi:10.1371/journal.pone.0081997. http://journals.plos.org/plosone/article?id=10.1371/journal.pone.0081997. Accessed on February 22, 2017.

McKirnan, D. J., et al. 2013. "Health Care Access and Health Behaviors among Men Who Have Sex with Men: The Cost of Health Disparities." *Public Health Education & Behavior*, 40(1): 32–41.

McQuillan, Geraldine, et al. 2017. "Prevalence of HPV in Adults Aged 18–69: United States, 2011–2014." Centers for Disease Control and Prevention. https://www.cdc.gov/nchs/products/databriefs/db280.htm. Accessed on April 9, 2017.

MMWR. 1996. "Summary of Notifiable Diseases, United States, 1995." *Morbidity and Mortality Weekly Report*. https://www.cdc.gov/mmwr/preview/mmwrhtml/00044418.htm. Accessed on March 4, 2017.

MMWR. 2001. "HIV and AIDS—United States, 1981–2000." *Morbidity and Mortality Weekly Report*. https://www.cdc.gov/mmwr/preview/mmwrhtml/mm5021a2.htm. Accessed on February 21, 2017.

National Cancer Institute (NCI)-Designated Cancer Centers. 2016. "NCI-Designated Cancer Centers Urge HPV Vaccination for the Prevention of Cancer." https://old.cancer.org/acs/groups/cid/@healthpromotions/documents/document/acspc-047188.pdf. Accessed on February 21, 2017.

National Coalition of STD Directors. 2016. "Funding Landscape." http://www.ncsddc.org/funding-landscape. Accessed on February 11, 2017.

National Coalition of STD Directors. n.d. "Impact of Sequestration on the Prevention of Sexually Transmitted Diseases." http://www.ncsddc.org/sites/default/files/final_sequestration_impact_on_std_prevention_0.pdf. Accessed on February 13, 2017.

National Conference of State Legislators. 2017. "HPV Vaccine: State Legislation and Statutes." http://www.ncsl.org/research/health/hpv-vaccine-state-legislation-and-statutes.aspx#. Accessed on February 18, 2017.

National Health Service [UK]. 2015. "Chlamydia—Complications." http://www.nhs.uk/Conditions/Chlamydia/Pages/Complications.aspx. Accessed on February 15, 2017.

National Institute of Allergy and Infectious Diseases. 2016. "NIAID Appropriations History: FY 2006–FY 2015." Fiscal Year 2015 Fact Book. https://www.niaid.nih.gov/sites/default/files/FY15Factbk.pdf. Accessed on February 11, 2017.

National Institutes of Health. 1996. "AIDS Vaccine Research Highlights." https://aidsinfo.nih.gov/news/282/aids-vaccine-research-highlights. Accessed on February 23, 2017.

National Institutes of Health. 2013. "Cervical Cancer." https://report.nih.gov/nihfactsheets/viewfactsheet.aspx?csid=76. Accessed on February 18, 2017.

National Institutes of Health. 2016a. "Large-Scale HIV Vaccine Trial to Launch in South Africa." https://www.nih.gov/news-events/news-releases/large-scale-hiv-vaccine-trial-launch-south-africa. Accessed on February 23, 2017.

National Institutes of Health. 2016b. "Trial of a Therapeutic DNA Vaccine for Chronic Hepatitis C Virus (HCV) Infection." https://clinicaltrials.gov/ct2/show/NCT02772003. Accessed on March 1, 2017.

Nelson, Roxanne. 2016. "HPV Vaccination Controversy in Japan, Rates Plummet to 1%." *Medscape*. http://www.medscape.com/viewarticle/866405. Accessed on February 20, 2017.

Newton, David E. 2013. *Vaccination Controversies: A Reference Handbook*. Santa Barbara, CA: ABC-CLIO.

Newson, Louise. 2015. "Cervical Cancer." *Patient*. http://patient.info/doctor/cervical-cancer-pro. Accessed on February 17, 2017.

North American Syringe Exchange Network. 2017. "Syringe Services Program Coverage in the United States—June 2014." https://nasen.org/site_media/files/amfar-sep-map/amfar-sep-map-2014.pdf. Accessed on February 26, 2017.

Nsnbc International. 2015. "Denmark drops Gardasil HPV Vaccine for Cervarix." https://nsnbc.me/2015/09/25/denmark-drops-gardasil-hpv-vaccine-for-cervarix/. Accessed on February 20, 2017.

Null, Gary. n.d. "HPV Vaccines: Unnecessary and Lethal." PRN.FM. http://prn.fm/gary-null-hpv-vaccines-unnecessary-and-lethal-2/. Accessed on February 20, 2017.

O'Leary, Dale. 2014. "The Syndemic of AIDS and STDS among MSM." *Linacre Quarterly*, 81(1): 12–37.

Ontario Harm Reduction Distribution Program. 2017. "Products for Safer Drugs Use." http://www.ohrdp.ca/products/. Accessed on February 26, 2017.

Page, Kimberly, et al. 2013. "Injection Drug Use and Hepatitis C Virus Infection in Young Adult Injectors: Using Evidence to Inform Comprehensive Prevention." *Clinical Infectious Diseases*, 57 (Suppl 2): S32–S38.

Perry, Rick. 2007. "Speech—May 8, 2007." http://www.lrl.state.tx.us/scanned/govdocs/Rick%20Perry/2007/remarks050807.pdf. Accessed on February 18, 2017.

Planned Parenthood. 2015. "2014–2015 Annual Report." https://www.plannedparenthood.org/files/2114/5089/0863/2014-2015_PPFA_Annual_Report_pdf. Accessed on March 7, 2017.

ProCon.org. 2017. "Should Any Vaccines Be Required for Children?" http://vaccines.procon.org/. Accessed on February 21, 2017.

Rerks-Ngarm, Supachai, et al. 2009. "Vaccination with ALVAC and AIDSVAX to Prevent HIV-1 Infection in Thailand." *New England Journal of Medicine*, 361(23): 2209-2220.

Rhode Island Center for Freedom and Prosperity. 2015. "The Debate about Rhode Island's HPV Vaccine Mandate (Draft)." http://rifreedom.org/wp-content/uploads/HPV-1-pager.pdf. Accessed on February 21, 2017.

Ruf, Murad, and Oliver Morgan. 2008. "Diagnosis and Screening: Differences between Screening and Diagnostic Tests, Case Finding." *Health Knowledge.* https://www.healthknowledge.org.uk/public-health-textbook/disease-causation-diagnostic/2c-diagnosis-screening/screening-diagnostic-case-finding. Accessed on February 16, 2017.

Ryerson, A. Blythe, et al. 2016. "Annual Report to the Nation on the Status of Cancer, 1975-2012, Featuring the Increasing Incidence of Liver Cancer." *Cancer*, 122(9): 1312–1337. http://onlinelibrary.wiley.com/doi/10.1002/cncr.29936/full. Accessed on February 18, 2017.

Sagonowsky, Eric. 2016. "GSK Exits US Market with Its HPV Vaccine Cervarix." *FiercePharma.* http://www.fiercepharma.com/pharma/gsk-exits-u-s-market-its-hpv-vaccine-cervarix. Accessed on February 18, 2017.

Scheel, Troels, K. H., et al. 2015. "Characterization of Nonprimate Hepacivirus and Construction of a Functional Molecular Clone." *Proceedings of the National Academy of Sciences*, 112(7): 2192-2197. http://www.pnas.org/content/112/7/2192.full. Accessed on March 1, 2017.

Schoenstadt, Arthur. 2017. "Types of HPV." eMedTV. http://hpv.emedtv.com/hpv/types-of-hpv.html. Accessed on February 17, 2017.

Schwartz, Pepper, and Martha Kempner. 2015. *50 Great Myths of Human Sexuality*. Chichester, West Sussex: Wiley-Blackwell.

Scott, Hyman M., and Jeffrey D. Klausner. 2016. "Sexually Transmitted Infections and Pre-exposure Prophylaxis: Challenges and Opportunities among Men Who Have Sex with Men in the US." *AIDS Research and Therapy*, 13(1). doi:10.1186/s12981-016-0089-8. https://aidsrestherapy.biomedcentral.com/articles/10.1186/s12981-016-0089-8. Accessed on February 22, 2017.

Scott, T. F. McNair. 1986. "Historical Aspects of Herpes Simplex Infections: Part 1." *International Journal of Dermatology*, 25(1): 63–70.

Sharma, Harsha, et al. 2014. "Microbiota and Pelvic Inflammatory Disease." *Seminars in Reproductive Medicine*, 32(1): 43–49. https://www.ncbi.nlm.nih.gov/pmc/articles/PMC4148456/. Accessed on November 7 2017.

Sheets, Rebecca L., TieQun Zhou, and Ivana Knezevic. 2016. "Review of Efficacy Trials of HIV-1/AIDS Vaccines and Regulatory Lessons Learned: A Review from a Regulatory Perspective." *Biologicals*, 44(2): 73–89.

Shilhavey, Brian. 2017. "New Gardasil Vaccine Guidelines from American Cancer Society Censors All Risks to Vaccine." *Health Impact News*. https://healthimpactnews.com/2016/new-gardasil-vaccine-guidelines-from-american-cancer-society-censors-all-risks-to-vaccine/. Accessed on February 20, 2017.

Spring, Lyba. 2013. "HPV Vaccine: Why Aren't Canadians Buying In?" *Canadian Women's Health Network*. http://

www.cwhn.ca/en/networkmagazine/hpvvaccinewhyarent
canadiansbuyingin?page=show. Accessed on February 20,
2017.

Stoner, Bradley P., and Stephanie E. Cohen. 2015.
"Lymphogranuloma Venereum 2015: Clinical Presentation,
Diagnosis, and Treatment." *Clinical Infectious Diseases*, 61
(Suppl 8): S865-S873. http://sfcityclinic.org/providers/
StonerBP_LGV.pdf. Accessed on March 5, 2017.

Substance Abuse and Mental Health Services Administration.
n.d. "Syringe Exchange Program Studies." http://archive.
samhsa.gov/ssp/docs/SyringeExchangeProgramStudies.pdf.
Accessed on March 1, 2017.

Taylor-Robinson, David, and Jørgen Skov Jensen. 2011.
"*Mycoplasma Genitalium*: from Chrysalis to Multicolored
Butterfly." *Clinical Microbiology Reviews*, 24(3): 498–514.

Thaler, Malcolm. 2015. "Men Get Yeast Infections, Too!"
One Medical. http://www.onemedical.com/blog/live-well/
male-yeast-infection/. Accessed on February 16, 2017.

Truong, H-H. M., et al. 2006. "Increases in Sexually
Transmitted Infections and Sexual Risk Behaviour without
a Concurrent Increase in HIV Incidence among Men Who
Have Sex with Men in San Francisco: A Suggestion of
HIV Serosorting?" *Sexually Transmitted Infections*, 82(6):
461–466.

Unemo, Magnus, and Robert A. Nicholas. 2012. "Emergence
of Multidrug-resistant, Extensively Drug-resistant and
Untreatable Gonorrhea." *Future Microbiology*, 7(12):
1401–1422. https://www.ncbi.nlm.nih.gov/pmc/articles/
PMC3629839/. Accessed on February 11, 2017.

U.S. Food and Drug Administration. 2006. "FDA Licenses
New Vaccine for Prevention of Cervical Cancer and Other
Diseases in Females Caused by Human Papillomavirus:
Rapid Approval Marks Major Advancement in Public
Health." https://www.fda.gov/NewsEvents/Newsroom/

PressAnnouncements/2006/ucm108666.htm. Accessed on February 18, 2017.

U.S. Food and Drug Administration. 2015. "The Drug Development Process." https://www.fda.gov/ForPatients/ Approvals/Drugs/default.htm. Accessed on March 1, 2017.

U.S. Military HIV Research Program. 2017. "RV144 Trial." http://www.hivresearch.org/rv144-trial. Accessed on February 23, 2017.

Van der Laar, et al. 2006. "A Slow Epidemic of LGV in the Netherlands in 2004 and 2005." *Eurosurveillance*, 11(7-9): 150–152.

Van Miert, A. S. J. P. A. M. 1994. "The Sulfonamide– Diaminopyrimidine Story." *Journal of Veterinary Pharmacology and Therapeutics*, 17(4): 309–316.

Vanderbilt University. 2017. "Key Health Concerns for WSW (Women Who Have Sex with Women)" and "Key Health Concerns for MSM (Men Who Have Sex with Men)." Program for LGBTI Health. https://medschool.vanderbilt. edu/lgbti/health-concerns-wsw. Accessed on February 14, 2017.

Vermont Coalition for Vaccine Choice. 2017. "Pro-Safety, Pro-Health. Vaccine Choice. It Is Your Inalienable Right to Decide!" http://www.vaxchoicevt.com/. Accessed on February 21, 2017.

Viborga, Ilze. 2006. "The Clinical Appearance of Pelvic Inflammatory Disease in Relation to Use of Intrauterine Device in Latvia." Uppsala Universitet. https://www.diva-portal.org/smash/get/diva2:167766/FULLTEXT01.pdf. Accessed on February 17, 2017.

WebMD. 2017. "The Basics about Genital Herpes." http:// www.webmd.com/genital-herpes/guide/genital-herpes-basics#1-3. Accessed on March 3, 2017.

White, Mark Donald. 2014. "Pros, Cons, and Ethics of HPV Vaccine in Teens—Why Such Controversy?" *Translational*

Andrology and Urology, 3(4): 429–434. https://www.ncbi.nlm.nih.gov/pmc/articles/PMC4708146/. Accessed on February 19, 2017.

Whittington, William L. H., et al. 2002. "Sexually Transmitted Diseases and Human Immunodeficiency Virus—Discordant Partnerships among Men Who Have Sex with Men." *Clinical Infectious Diseases*, 35(8): 1010-1017. https://academic.oup.com/cid/article/35/8/1010/328729/Sexually-Transmitted-Diseases-and-Human. Accessed on February 14, 2017.

Workowski, Kimberly A., and Gail A. Bolan. 2015. "Sexually Transmitted Diseases Treatment Guidelines, 2015." *Morbidity and Mortality Weekly*, 64(RR3): 1–137.

World Cancer Research Fund International. 2015. "Cervical Cancer Statistics." http://www.wcrf.org/int/cancer-facts-figures/data-specific-cancers/cervical-cancer-statistics. Accessed on February 18, 2017.

World Health Organization. 2012. "Global Action Plan to Control the Spread and Impact of Antimicrobial Resistance in *Neisseria gonorrhoeae*." Geneva: World Health Organization. http://apps.who.int/iris/bitstream/10665/44863/1/9789241503501_eng.pdf. Accessed on February 11, 2017.

World Health Organization. 2016a. Hepatitis Fact Sheets. http://www.who.int/mediacentre/factsheets/fs328/en/, http://www.who.int/mediacentre/factsheets/fs204/en/, and http://www.who.int/mediacentre/factsheets/fs164/en/. Accessed on February 25, 2017.

World Health Organization. 2016b. "Sexually Transmitted Infections." http://www.who.int/mediacentre/factsheets/fs110/en/. Accessed on February 15, 2017.

Zur Hausen, Harald. 2009. "Papillomaviruses in the Causation of Human Cancers—A Brief Historical Account." *Virology*, 384(2): 260–265.

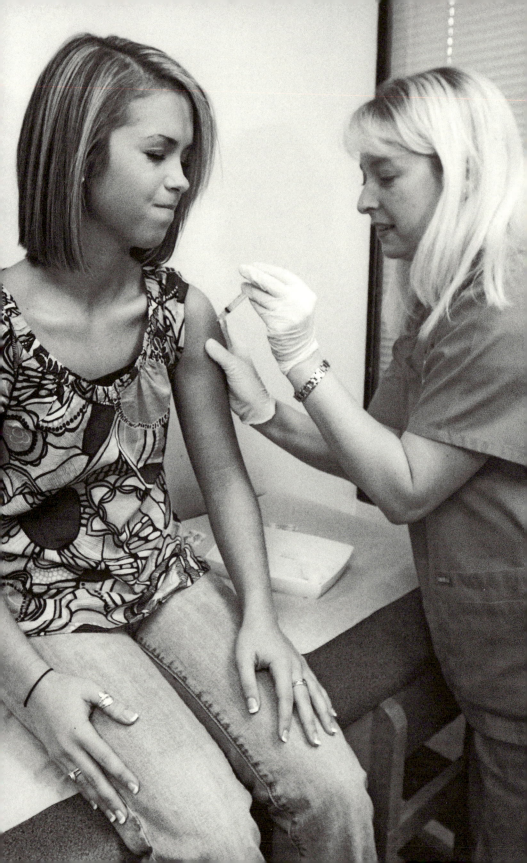

Introduction

The purpose of this chapter is to provide an opportunity to interested parties who would like to write more about some specific aspect of the topic of sexually transmitted infections (STIs). Thus you will find essays on the nature and value of syringe exchange programs (Alsum), expedited partner therapy (Choat), successful STI prevention programs (Ferrer), the experience of a pap smear (Herlihy), the stigma that sometimes surrounds STIs (Paluzzi), special issues involving STIs during pregnancy (Shannon), economic aspects of human papillomavirus (HPV) vaccination programs (Tsang), and condom negotiation (Nydegger). These essays provide an overview of the wide range of issues that can arise in any discussion of STIs.

Syringe Access and HIV
Stephen Alsum

Syringe access programs, while often portrayed in the media as controversial, are just good solid public health practice. At their most basic level, syringe access programs provide people with access to the tools they need to stay alive. For people suffering from the disease of addiction and injecting drugs, one of

A teenage girl winces as she receives the third and final application of the human papillomavirus (HPV) vaccine. (AP Photo/John Amis)

131

the tools needed to protect their health, and that of their community, is a sterile syringe.

Historically, in the United States, drug use has been met through the framework of either prevention or treatment. Prevention can be loosely defined as keeping people from using drugs in the first place and treatment as helping people to completely abstain from any and all drug use. The problem with addressing drug use from only these two modalities is that there is an incredible amount of middle ground in between prevention and treatment: the space after people have initiated drug use yet before they are ready to completely and totally abstain. In this middle ground, people still have need of health-related resources to help reduce the potential harms of their drug use, to themselves, and to their communities.

Harm reduction arose as a strategy to address this middle ground between prevention and treatment. Harm reduction can be loosely defined as a set of practical strategies aimed at reducing negative impacts of drug use. Harm reduction programs meet people where they are at; they do not expect people to make changes in their lives that they are not yet ready to make. Harm reduction programs present a range of options for how a client can improve his or her health; it is up to the client to choose which option will fit best with his or her life circumstances. These programs are also low threshold and accessible. A good metaphor to explain harm reduction relates to automobiles. Historically, automobile accidents have been the leading cause of accidental deaths in the United States. Driving an automobile is a potentially very dangerous behavior, even deadly, that many of us still engage in. Yet when we drive in automobiles, we take small steps to reduce the potential harm that could come to us and others from this behavior. We do things like wearing our seat belts, stopping at red lights, and driving reasonably within the speed limit. These are all ways that we are practicing harm reduction when we drive in cars. When addressing the danger of automobile accidents, we do not expect people to just stop driving in cars. Rather, practical options are presented to reduce the potential harm of that behavior. Likewise, in the midst of the HIV epidemic, where are our seat belts for drug use?

One of the potential harms that can come from drug use, and specifically injection drug use, is the transmission of HIV. HIV can be transmitted through blood-to-blood contact. Through injection drug use, this happens when people share syringes and other injection supplies. In our society, we have criminalized many forms of drug use, and in many locations, we have criminalized the implements people use to take drugs, including syringes. What this often leads to is a lack of access to syringes, which leads to people sharing syringes, which can lead to the transmission of HIV, and other blood-borne viruses such as hepatitis C. For most people who inject drugs, if they have access to sterile syringes, they will use them; however, if they do not have access, they will still continue their drug use albeit using a used syringe. The issue is not behavioral, it is structural; provided that we change the structure of our society so that sterile syringes are more accessible, most people's behaviors will naturally change and they will use sterile syringes. Hence the advent of syringe access programs.

Syringe access programs arose in the early 1990s as a response to rising rates of HIV infection among people who inject drugs, their families, and their friends. Since that time, syringe access programs have been highly studied in the scientific literature. Studies have found, over and over again, that syringe access programs are an effective, and furthermore cost-effective, means to prevent the spread of HIV, and that they can actually tend to reduce community levels of drug use. By providing access to sterile syringes, syringe access programs have been shown to decrease HIV in communities by up to 80 percent (Des Jarlais, Arasteh, and Friedman 2011). They also save an incredible amount of taxpayer dollars. While individual syringes can cost less the 50 cents to distribute, the average lifetime cost of treating HIV can range from $385,200 to $618,900 (Schackman et al. 2006). Studies have found that syringe access programs not only do not encourage drug use, but they can actually help people access treatment, with program participants being five times more likely to access treatment than non-participants (Hagan et al. 2000). Although our public discourse often focuses on the controversy of syringe access, an informed observer realizes they are just good solid public health.

Finally, syringe access fits snuggly within the confines of human rights and social justice. The means and the tools to protect our health should be a basic human right. For people who inject drugs, one of these tools is a sterile syringe. In our society, we have criminalized the disease of drug addiction, and often the person using the drug suffers. By the very nature of criminalization, there is extreme social stigma around drug use, serving to marginalize the person using drugs. A secondary benefit of syringe access programs includes providing a warm and welcoming environment in which people can be open and honest about who they are and where they are in their lives, something every human being needs.

References

Des Jarlais, D. C., K. Arasteh, and S. R. Friedman. 2011. "HIV among Drug Users at Beth Israel Medical Center, New York City, the First 25 Years." *Substance Use & Misuse*, 46(2–3): 131–139.

Hagan H., et al. 2000. "Reduced Injection Frequency and Increased Entry and Retention in Drug Treatment Associated with Needle-Exchange Participation in Seattle Drug Injectors." *Journal of Substance Abuse Treatment*, 19: 247–252.

Schackman, B. R., et al. 2006. "The Lifetime Cost of Current Human Immunodeficiency Virus Care in the United States." *Medical Care*, 44(11): 990–997.

Stephen Alsum holds a BS in Mathematics from Grand Valley State University and is the executive director of the Grand Rapids Red Project, a not-for-profit organization with the mission to improve health, reduce risk, and prevent HIV.

Expedited Partner Therapy and the Role It Can Play in Reducing Sexually Transmitted Infections
Lesli Choat

Treating sex partners of patients diagnosed with chlamydia and/or gonorrhea without physical examination by a health care provider is known as expedited partner therapy (EPT). The clinician provides either prescriptions or medications to the patient to be given to his/her sex partners (Centers for Disease Control and Prevention, Arizona State University 2011). EPT can be effective in reducing the spread of sexually transmitted infections (STIs) by preventing re-infections, reducing the numbers of infections within a community, and decreasing the number of complications young females experience from untreated STIs. EPT can mean the difference of each partner receiving treatment or being left untreated.

In 2015, the total number of chlamydia and gonorrhea cases was the highest ever reported in the United States (totaling 1,526,658 and 395,216, respectively; U.S. Department of Health and Human Services, Centers for Disease Control and Prevention 2015). Two-thirds of the cases of chlamydia and gonorrhea occur in individuals under the age of 25. For the last several years, the STIs have been increasing at an alarming rate costing health care approximately $16 billion annually. It is estimated that each year in the United States, there are 20 million new STIs and more than 110 million existing cases (U.S. Department of Health and Human Services, Centers for Disease Control and Prevention 2015). EPT must be considered when looking at ways to combat the rising rates of STIs.

Due to the asymptomatic nature of many STIs, the patient and partner are likely unaware of their infection and therefore do not seek treatment. However, those diagnosed with chlamydia or gonorrhea can easily be treated and cured with antibiotics. It is crucial that all partners are treated to avoid reinfection and further spread. Reinfection rates can be as high as 25 percent especially in adolescent females who can face serious complications from chlamydia and gonorrhea such as pelvic inflammatory disease (PID), ectopic pregnancy, or even infertility (Gaydos et al. 2008).

Partner services is notification, testing, and treatment of partners to patients diagnosed with an STI and is an essential part of STI prevention. Traditional methods of partner services are central for syphilis and HIV case management but are marginally effective for chlamydia and gonorrhea for several reasons. First, partner services is labor intensive and costly especially when faced with the large volume of chlamydia/gonorrhea infections. Second, partner services is dependent on state and county local health departments, most of which have suffered budget cuts and loss of staff over the past several years. And finally, many barriers exist that make it difficult for a partner to seek/obtain services (such as confidentiality, anger and shame, failure to acknowledge infection due to lack of symptoms, transportation, and lack of insurance or fear of using insurance when an explanation of benefit services might be sent to the parent).

Optimal partner services would be to have every partner seen by a clinician to receive testing and treatment for possible infections, but as shown, that is not always possible. EPT is also referred to as patient-delivered partner treatment (PDPT); sex partners (within the previous 60 days) of patients testing positive for certain STIs are provided treatment without medical evaluation (Centers for Disease Control and Prevention 2006). When medications for EPT are provided for sex partners, they should be accompanied by a written treatment instruction fact sheet. Written instructions should include appropriate warnings about taking medications and possible side effects (if the partner is pregnant or has an allergy to the medication), a statement encouraging partners to seek medical evaluation (especially if a more serious infection is suspected), and recommendation the partner be re-screened for STIs in three months. EPT is not routinely recommended for pregnant women, men who have sex with men (MSM), or in cases of suspected child abuse (Centers for Disease Control and Prevention 2006). EPT should be administered in accordance with current STD treatment guidelines of the Centers for Disease Control and Prevention (CDC), and dual therapy (two antibiotics given at the same time) must be used to treat all cases for gonorrhea (Centers for Disease Control and Prevention 2015). Risk for serious adverse reaction is quite low for the regimens recommended for use as EPT (Centers for Disease Control and Prevention 2006).

EPT has been considered the standard of care since the CDC recommendation in 2006. Numerous medical and professional organizations have issued statements of support, including American Medical Association, American Bar Association, Society for Adolescent Medicine, American Academy of Pediatrics, National Association of City and County Health Officials, American Congress of Obstetricians and Gynecologists Committee, and National Coalition of STD Directors.

As of December 2016, EPT is legal in 38 states (Centers for Disease Control and Prevention 2016). EPT rules differ slightly depending on state and can be found by selecting the state name at the CDC website https://www.cdc.gov/std/ept/. Some state guidelines include trichomoniasis as an STI that can be treated using EPT, and some states do not allow EPT for treating gonorrhea cases.

EPT is often underutilized because patients and clinicians are not aware of it. Some clinicians are not comfortable using EPT even though not treating partners is significantly more harmful than is the use of EPT. Be informed. If you are diagnosed with an STI, ask your provider about EPT. It is possible to access EPT services at many local health departments, community health centers, Planned Parenthood sites, some primary care physicians, and youth centers offering sexual health services.

References

Centers for Disease Control and Prevention. 2006.
  "Expedited Partner Therapy in Management of Sexually
  Transmitted Diseases." https://www.cdc.gov/std/treatment/
  eptfinalreport2006.pdf. Accessed on March 8, 2017.

Centers for Disease Control and Prevention. 2015. "Sexually Transmitted Diseases Treatment Guidelines." *Morbidity and Mortality Weekly Report*, 64(3). https://www.cdc.gov/std/tg2015/tg-2015-print.pdf. Accessed on March 8, 2017.

Centers for Disease Control and Prevention. 2016. "Legal Status of EPT." https://www.cdc.gov/std/ept/legal/default.htm. Accessed on March 8, 2017.

Centers for Disease Control and Prevention, Arizona State University. 2011. "Legal/Policy Toolkit for Adoption and Implementation of Expedited Partner Therapy." https://www.cdc.gov/std/ept/legal/ept-toolkit-complete.pdf. Accessed on March 8, 2017.

Gaydos, C. A., et al. 2008. "Chlamydia trachomatis Reinfection Rates among Female Adolescents Seeking Rescreening in School-Based Health Centers." *Sexually Transmitted Diseases*, 35(3): 233–237.

U.S. Department of Health and Human Services, Centers for Disease Control and Prevention. 2015. "Sexually Transmitted Disease Surveillance." https://www.cdc.gov/std/stats15/std-surveillance-2015-print.pdf. Accessed on March 8, 2017.

Lesli Choat holds a Bachelor of Science degree and has been a Board Certified Medical Technologist through the American Society for Clinical Pathologists (ASCP) since 1985. She has been employed in state government, public health since 1995 in both the Division of Laboratories and the Division of Infectious Disease. In 2012, she assumed the titles of STD counseling and testing coordinator and viral hepatitis prevention coordinator.

Using Public Transportation to Increase Awareness of Syphilis
Josh Ferrer

"So what exactly is this campaign going to be about?" the transit advertising representative sitting across from me asked.

"Syphilis," I replied. Without batting an eye, she scribbled on her notepad and I proceeded to tell her more. By the end of our conversation, she had the common reaction of most people when told that Oregon is in the middle of a syphilis epidemic. "I had no idea it was such a problem," she said.

As recently as late 1990s, there was talk nationally about eradicating syphilis. The number of cases had dropped to historically low levels and the Centers for Disease Control and Prevention (CDC) launched a national initiative to eliminate new cases (Centers for Disease Control and Prevention 2010).

However, syphilis is a formidable opponent, and like many other states, Oregon began to experience a resurgence of cases in the mid-2000s. From 2007 to 2015, rates of the two earliest and most infectious stages of syphilis (primary and secondary) increased over 1,500% across the state (Sexually Transmitted Infections in Oregon 2016). The majority of cases occurred in and around Portland, the largest city in Oregon, among gay, bisexual and other men who have sex with men.

In 2013, the Oregon Public Health Division and the Multnomah County Health Department, which encompasses Portland, requested assistance from the CDC in order to gain a greater understanding of why syphilis was continuing to increase. By January 2014, behavioral and social scientists from CDC had come to Portland to conduct a variety of projects including interviews with health care providers, HIV/STD prevention outreach workers, and members of the community who were at risk for acquiring syphilis or who had it in the past. Among the findings was that men were unaware that syphilis was a serious problem, or believed it was no big deal. Additionally, men reported confusion over signs and symptoms of syphilis, mistaking them for other STDs such as herpes or gonorrhea, as well as confusion over what a test for syphilis involved. In their list of recommendations for future action, CDC scientists recommended consideration of a multilevel social marketing campaign to inform men that syphilis was an issue and to make them aware of signs, symptoms, and testing options.

In the spring of 2015, staff in the Oregon Public Health Division STD program considered a variety of options to inform the public and medical providers about the syphilis epidemic. While the epidemic was concentrated in men having sex with men in the Portland–Metro area, we were continuing to see a number of other cases statewide, and disconcertingly, our syphilis rates among women had been doubling year to year with a handful of congenital (mother-to-child) cases.

The idea of a transit campaign was one of many being tossed around. The Portland area has the enviable reputation of having an excellent and widely used transit system of buses and light rail. What if we were to advertise on the sides and backs of buses and trains with some ads on the ceiling thrown in for good measure? We knew that focusing the campaign solely around men would only have partial impact. The ads would be too easy for many people to tune out, thinking "that doesn't impact me." The desire was strong to have a campaign that did not just target gay men, but also their best friends, grandmothers, and other people who care about them. We also knew that we wanted to target medical providers and they ride mass transit or drive and see buses all the time just like everyone else.

Thus the campaign we had dubbed SyphAware began to take off. We message tested a variety of slogans with partners and members of the community and arrived at the following winning message:

Portland

Nationally we're. . .

#1 for coffee

#1 for fitness

#5 for syphilis

Get Informed. SyphAware.org

This message seemed to resonate most because it was both surprising and thought-provoking. It contrasted many of the things most positively associated with Portland, including its superb coffee and health-conscious level of fitness, with the knowledge that from 2009 to 2013 the greater Portland area was tied for fifth nationally in primary and secondary syphilis among the 50 most populous metropolitan statistical areas (Centers for Disease Control and Prevention 2014).

An advertising firm then took our slogans along with a diverse array of stock image models and created a variety of ads that appeared on buses and train cars. Over 115 ads ran, beginning in November 2015. Attention from the media accompanying the launch of the first ads was immediate with multiple stories appearing quickly on TV and radio and in newspapers. The campaign gained national attention and went viral a few months later when the same model used for some of the ads also appeared in an ad for a group supporting Hillary Clinton's presidential campaign. A second wave of the campaign appeared on over 100 buses in Eugene, Oregon, in November 2016.

To make sure that people had access to concise and accurate information in an eye-catching way, we worked with designers to create a campaign website (SyphAware). The site contains basic information on signs and symptoms, testing options, preventing syphilis, and an interactive quiz where folks can test their syphilis knowledge and learn if more routine screening is right for them.

Time will tell whether the SyphAware campaign has had any sort of measurable impact, and we continue to work on evaluation activities to see whether screening patterns among medical providers and the public have shifted. It was a relatively small campaign given our limited resources but it garnered a great deal of media attention and has inspired conversations in the community. Ultimately, on that point alone it can be considered a success. Silence, discomfort, and a lack of conversation around sexual health and STDs like syphilis only continue to contribute to their spread. Who knows? Hopefully the campaign inspired a few grandmothers to talk to their grandkids about that ad they saw on the side of the bus.

References

Centers for Disease Control and Prevention. 2010. "Syphilis Elimination Effort." https://www.cdc.gov/stopsyphilis/. Accessed March 27, 2017.

Centers for Disease Control and Prevention. 2014. "Sexually Transmitted Disease Surveillance 2013." https://www.cdc.gov/std/stats13/surv2013-print.pdf. Accessed on April 1, 2017.

"Sexually Transmitted Infections in Oregon: Everything You Wanted to Know." 2016. CD Summary, 65(1): 2–3.

"SyphAware." Oregon Health Authority. http://www.syphaware.org/. Accessed March 31, 2017.

Josh Ferrer is the HIV/STD technical consultant with the Oregon Public Health Division. He holds an MA degree from Miami University of Ohio and has worked in the field of HIV/STD prevention for over 10 years.

A New Era in the Stirrups
Stacy Mintzer Herlihy

It's a rite of passage for all young women: the first visit to the OB-GYN. For the first time in her life, a young woman will sit on the cold straps as someone probes the interior of her body. For most women, it's also the stuff of fierce and embedded memory, a time when they enter that classic experience that will be theirs for as long as they are adult women. I remember the terror and the fear and final sense of relief that it over far sooner than I had anticipated and I could put my own clothing on again in the cold white office. Every so often, every woman knows she will visit an OB to make sure nothing is growing where it should not. After the examination is completed with an internal probe and a pap smear, most women know they might get a call a few days later to let them know something's wrong. Most women will grow used to the wait. For some, the news will be confirmation of an existing problem or the creation of a new one. Many women will relax periodically reassured that's nothing gone wrong yet.

I've never gotten that call. I've been lucky. I have never known the hell of a bad pap and all that comes with it.

For a new generation, this ritual in the stirrups is now a whole lot easier and will be a lot less stressful going forward. The reason is an exciting and highly effective vaccine. For so many of us, HPV is an entirely new collection of letters that had not been part of our lives. The only time I'd ever heard of it was on an episode of *The West Wing*. The president's secretary was begging a researcher to find a way to cure or prevent the virus because her sister had died from the disease. I listened, puzzled, and gave it no other thought for many years. HPV stands for human papillomavirus. The letters also stand for the HPV vaccine. Researchers have long sought to find a vaccine. The vaccine has been highly tested, checked, and then checked again and then finally brought to market. Today, it's part of standard health care for women in many countries.

In many ways, the creation of the vaccine has been a revelation. For many of us, the vaccine meant suddenly hearing about a disease that had been in the shadows but wasn't really in the shadows at all. After the vaccine became part of the conversation, friends suddenly told me of their struggles with HPV infection, stories they had only hinted at before. My best friend confided the deeply sad tale of her sister stricken with a serious HPV infection in her early thirties and horrified at the life choices it presented her with. The infection was so bad she ultimately had to have a hysterectomy at the age of 32. Others told me of their own mothers or sisters or aunts infected with a miserable thing that ate at body parts and make each pap smear something to be dreaded for weeks afterward. I asked my own OB about the vaccine. He told me he was grateful he could now offer the vaccine to his patients. Time and again he had watched as his patients had dealt with the frustrating and ugly aftereffects of an infection. The new vaccine would help vastly reduce his patient's pain, decrease the risk of cancer, and make pregnancies safer.

A Common Infection

Once the vaccine has come to the forefront, many of us have learned that it is surprisingly common. Nearly all of us, men and women alike, will get infected with one form of HPV or another during the course of our lives. Most of us will have no problem with it and never need to think about these three letters again. The infection will pass through our system without our even knowing about it. Yet, for millions of others, the virus may cause horrible side effects. Millions of people will get genital warts or even any one of several kinds of cancers as a friend of mine found out when she had to get treatment for the HPV-caused cancer that had spread to the base of her tongue. The great news is that this doesn't have to be this way going forward. Teenagers today can get three doses of the vaccine before they are 15. As a result, any teen today, female and male, will face a much lower risk of being infected with a nasty disease that might otherwise haunt his or her life.

As the mother of two daughters, the new vaccine delights me. My eldest child has already gotten the required three doses. She, as so many others in this country and all over the world, can now look forward to the protection of the vaccine. Instead of her first pap smear, she will likely face a world in which she will have a test for HPV infection. Should the test prove negative, she may be spared the ritual of the yearly pap smear and all the fear that goes with it. Hers will likely be a world where many forms of cancer from cervical cancer to vulva cancers are far less common. In her world, there will be fewer whispered stories of the sudden realization that a hysterectomy was necessary before she's even graduated from college. In her world, genital warts may be a rare thing, and changes in her cervix that might signal something is wrong will also be ever more rare.

This is the world that I hope she and her peers will find themselves part of forever: a place where that rite of passage is a lot less scary and a lot less potentially dangerous. I hope that she and her peers will not know what life was like before the vaccine, when women worried every single time they put on that robe and steered their legs into the cold metal stirrups.

Stacy Mintzer Herlihy is a freelance writer based in New Jersey and the mother of two daughters. She is the coauthor of Your Baby's Best Shot: Why Vaccines Are Safe and Save Lives.

Stigma and STIs
Patricia Paluzzi

Sexually transmitted infections (STIs), also called sexually transmitted diseases, have been around for centuries. Syphilis is one of the oldest recorded STIs, and both famous and infamous people of their day such as Henry VIII, Beethoven, Al Capone, Napoleon, and, apparently, even Honest Abe Lincoln suffered from this most damaging disease. They did not have proper treatment available to them, and some of them ultimately died from side effects of syphilis, but we do not have to suffer the same fate. We know so much more know about all kinds of STIs that there is only one reason someone might have long-term problems because of an STI—shame!

The stigma and shame associated with having an STI were there in the beginning and have persisted over time preventing many of us, young and old, from doing what we can to prevent getting an STI or seeking treatment. But what are we really worried about? Someone finding out? Being labeled in a negative way? Stigma and shame can cause a lot of harm because they may prevent us from doing what we know is best for us and our relationships.

So why is it so important to overcome one's shame about STIs? Well for one thing, young people account for almost half of all STIs in the United States. If you are having sex, then you can get an STI; it is that simple. Over 30 different "bugs" cause the various STIs we know about today. We have cures for most, treatments to reduce side effects of others, and can even prevent some with vaccinations. We know most are transmitted through sexual contact and that there are safer sex practices that can help us avoid getting infected, including abstinence and regular condom use.

If we don't get treated, some STIs can cause longer-term and more severe problems. For example, if left untreated, gonorrhea can cause infections that affect other parts of our body, HPV (venereal warts) is the leading cause of cervical cancer and is totally preventable with a vaccine, hepatitis B and C can impair other vital organs, and HIV and syphilis can cause death. And finally, we can harm someone else if we don't get treated by passing on an STI, many of which don't have symptoms. Scary stuff and sometimes being scared gets in the way of our seeking care, but it doesn't have to be scary because we live in a time when prevention and treatment are available.

There are a lot of resources available to help you understand STIs—what they are, when you should get tested, all about prevention, and much, much more. Health care providers are sworn to confidentiality, so you can discuss any of your concerns with them, and they won't tell anyone—and they won't judge you. It is really important that you are able to talk with your boy- or girlfriend about STIs, getting tested, using condoms, and so on. Scarlateen.org is a website for youth that is filled with a lot of sex ed information, and Sexetc.org is another site loaded with sex ed information that is written by teens for teens.

Healthy Teen Network is a national organization that provides resources to professionals who work with young people, especially regarding their sexual and reproductive health.

Healthy Teen Network provides support for creating clinics that are youth friendly, provides effective and comprehensive sex education in schools and after-school settings, addresses issues of racism and homophobism, and stresses the importance of considering where one lives, learns, and plays when promoting healthy behaviors.

In addition, Healthy Teen Network offers resources for young people that can be viewed alone or with a parent, guardian, or other caring adult. Go to www.healthyteennetwork.org and check out the following:

- *Keep It Simple*, a short film you can view alone or with an adult who can help you decide how best to manage your sexual health.
- *No Te Compliques*, *Keep It Simple* in Spanish
- VOLT, a series of resources you can view alone or with a caring adult who can help you assess your health needs and prepare for a visit with a clinician.
- CRUSHapp.org, is a web-based app intended for 15- to 17-year-old females but useful for anyone interested in learning more about how to decide if you are ready for sex, if your partner is a keeper, how contraception works, choosing one that is right with you, and finding a clinical provider.

Don't let stigma and shame keep you from being your best self. Be informed, take action, and be safe.

Patricia Paluzzi, CNM, DrPH, is president and CEO of Healthy Teen Network. She has been active in the fields of reproductive and maternal and child health for over 40 years, as a clinician, researcher, administrator, and advocate. Her clinical and content expertise spans the full scope of midwifery care, substance abuse, intimate partner violence, high-risk maternal child health (including pregnant teens), incorporating men into clinical services, and trauma-informed approaches.

Pregnancy and Sexually Transmitted Infections: A Missed Opportunity for Prevention
Chelsea Shannon

Every year, there are an estimated 357 million new infections with *Chlamydia trachomatis* (chlamydia), *Neisseria gonorrhoeae* (gonorrhea), *Trichomonas vaginalis* (trichomoniasis), or syphilis worldwide (World Health Organization 2016). In pregnant women, these bacterial infections can cause an increased risk of adverse birth outcomes or even infant death. Although the number of screening programs for maternal syphilis is growing, very few countries have any maternal screening programs in place for more common sexually transmitted infections (STIs) such as chlamydia, gonorrhea, or trichomoniasis. As rapid diagnostic tests for these STIs become increasingly available, corresponding prenatal screening programs should be implemented alongside prenatal syphilis screening programs around the world.

The World Health Organization (WHO) estimates 131 million new chlamydial infections, 78 million new gonococcal infections, 142 million new trichomonal infections, and 6 million new syphilis infections every year (World Health Organization 2016). However, rates of infection vary significantly by country and by demographic characteristics. STI rates in pregnant women are often above national rates, as young adults typically carry the highest burden of infection (Dehne and Riedner 2005).

Syphilis infection during pregnancy can cause severe adverse birth outcomes. Specifically, maternal syphilis has been associated with spontaneous abortion, stillbirth, premature labor, and other complications. If a woman transmits the infection to her fetus, causing congenital syphilis, the infant is at high risk of serious complications including brain and nerve problems, deformed bones, enlarged liver, and meningitis. Up to 40 percent of cases of untreated maternal syphilis infections lead to stillbirth or infant death (Congenital Syphilis 2017).

Chlamydia, gonorrhea, and trichomoniasis during pregnancy have also been linked to adverse birth outcomes, including premature labor and low birth weight infants. Furthermore, if the mother has an untreated chlamydial or gonococcal infection during birth, there is a 30-70 percent chance the infection will be passed to the infant. This could lead to eye infection and chlamydial pneumonitis in the case of chlamydia, or eye infection and blindness in the case of gonorrhea. Long-term untreated chlamydial or gonococcal infection in a woman can lead to pelvic inflammatory disease, which could cause future ectopic pregnancies, spontaneous abortion, or infertility. Finally, a woman with any of those infections is more likely to acquire HIV and, if HIV positive, more likely to transmit HIV to her baby (Adachi et al. 2015).

Chlamydia, gonorrhea, trichomoniasis, and syphilis are all bacterial infections, which means they can be cured with antibiotics. If a pregnant woman is screened and tests positive for one or more of these STIs, antibiotic treatment will cure the infection. Multiple studies have shown that antibiotic treatment of a bacterial STI during pregnancy significantly reduces the risk of adverse birth outcomes (McGregor et al. 1990; Temmerman et al. 1995). However, because many of these infections are usually without symptoms, prenatal screening programs are critical to diagnosis and treatment.

WHO currently recommends prenatal screening for syphilis, and has made the reduction of mother-to-child transmission of syphilis a priority in its Sustainable Development Goals (World Health Organization 2016). However, WHO provides no current recommendations for prenatal screening of other STIs such as chlamydia, gonorrhea, or trichomoniasis. For those STIs, WHO simply recommends symptom-based treatment. This is an inadequate approach, as many cases, especially in women, do not show any symptoms. Ten countries—the Bahamas, Bulgaria, Canada, Estonia, Japan, Germany, Democratic People's Republic of Korea, Romania, Sweden, and the United Kingdom—do recommend screening for these infections during pregnancy (Medline, Davey, and Klausner 2016). Others, such as the

United States, recommend screening pregnant women who are under the age of 25 or deemed to be at high risk for infection. Still, the majority of countries provide no prenatal screening recommendations for chlamydia, gonorrhea, or trichomoniasis.

The primary reason so many countries do not screen for STIs is not a lack of awareness but the high cost of screening. The current standard way to diagnose chlamydia, gonorrhea, or trichomoniasis is through nucleic acid amplification tests. That type of test requires a laboratory with machinery and trained personnel, and it typically takes multiple days to receive results. It is not a realistic option for many prenatal clinics around the world. To compare, syphilis screening can be done through rapid diagnostic tests that simply require a drop of blood and take less than 20 minutes to provide results.

Fortunately, many rapid diagnostic tests for STIs such as chlamydia, gonorrhea, and trichomoniasis are currently under development (Herbst de Cortina et al. 2016). Those tests will change the landscape of STI screening globally, as it will be quicker, simpler, and significantly less expensive to run screening tests. As rapid diagnostic tests become more readily available, the global health community must make it a priority to increase STI screening efforts, especially among pregnant women.

One of WHO's Sustainable Development Goals is to reduce neonatal mortality (World Health Organization 2016). Implementing prenatal STI screening programs around the world would likely lead to a significant reduction in adverse birth outcomes and infant mortality. Furthermore, maternal screening programs could pave the way for broader STI prevention programs in the future. With the advent of new rapid diagnostic tests, that will be more feasible than ever.

References

Adachi, Kristina, et al. 2015. "Chlamydia and Gonorrhea in HIV-Infected Pregnant Women and Infant HIV Transmission." *Sexually Transmitted Diseases*, 42(10): 554–565.

"Congenital Syphilis." 2017. CDC Fact Sheet. https://www. cdc.gov/std/syphilis/stdfact-congenital-syphilis.htm. Accessed on March 13, 2017.

Dehne, Karl L., and Gabriele Riedner. 2005. "Sexually Transmitted Infections among Adolescents. The Need for Adequate Health Services." World Health Organization. http://apps.who.int/iris/ bitstream/10665/43221/1/9241562889.pdf. Accessed on April 1, 2017.

Herbst de Cortina S., et al. 2016. "A Systematic Review of Point of Care Testing for Chlamydia Trachomatis, Neisseria Gonorrhoeae, and Trichomonas Vaginalis." *Infectious Diseases in Obstetrics and Gynecology.* doi:10.1155/2016/4386127.

McGregor, James A., et al. 1990. "Cervicovaginal Microflora and Pregnancy Outcome: Results of a Double-Blind, Placebo-Controlled Trial of Erythromycin Treatment." *American Journal of Obstetrics and Gynecology*, 163(5): 1580-1591.

Medline, Alexandra, Dvora Joseph Davey, and Jeffrey D. Klausner. 2016. "Lost Opportunity to Save Newborn Lives: Variable National Antenatal Screening Policies for Neisseria gonorrhoeae and Chlamydia trachomatis." *International Journal of STD & AIDS.* doi:09564624166604.

Temmerman, Marleen, et al. 1995. "Mass Antimicrobial Treatment in Pregnancy: A Randomized Placebo-Controlled Trial in a Population with High Rates of Sexually Transmitted Disease." *The Journal of Reproductive Medicine*, 40(3): 176–180.

World Health Organization. 2016. "Global Health Sector Strategy on Sexually Transmitted Infections, 2016-2021." http://apps.who.int/iris/bitstream/10665/246296/1/ WHO-RHR-16.09-eng.pdf. Accessed on April 2, 2017.

Chelsea Shannon works for the Division of Infectious Disease at the UCLA David Geffen School of Medicine. Her research interests include HIV, STI diagnostics, and STIs in pregnancy. Chelsea graduated from Stanford University and currently plans to pursue a career in medicine and global public health.

Economic Coverage of HPV Vaccination
Mia Tsang

In the exploration and investigation of sexually transmitted diseases, there will always be one name that consistently resurfaces: HPV, or human papillomavirus. This virus has been proven to be the principal cause of cervical cancer in women, but it can also cause penile cancer in men and anal cancer in both, as well as genital warts and a host of other non-lethal but still unpleasant side effects.

Recent years have brought about the development of several vaccines to combat HPV and, in turn, cervical cancer. However, there is a significant amount of controversy surrounding these vaccines. Parents worry that the vaccine may serve as a "potential gateway to encouraging sexual contact at earlier ages or promoting higher risk sexual practices"; essentially, once they are protected against HPV, teens may experience a false sense of security and start having sex earlier than they might have if they hadn't received the vaccine. They have also expressed the usual concerns that arise among parents with any vaccine: dangerous side effects and lack of efficacy to justify administration. This is where the majority of the controversy surrounding these vaccines has come from. But in the midst of the uproar, a vital part of this argument has flown largely under the radar: money.

The decision of who will pay for vaccine administration may be a less-publicized debate, but it is no less of a critical one. There are two main points: First, which type of vaccine should be covered? Second, should coverage be expanded across the board or should expansion be focused on specific regions of the country? It is imperative that one takes a look at these points from an economic standpoint, because if funds are allocated in the most efficient way, not only will the instance of disease occurrence decrease, but also more funds will be available to allocate for research into this disease and others.

There are three main HPV vaccines on the market: Gardasil (4vHPV), Ceravix (2vHPV), and Gardasil-9 (9vHPV). Gardasil-9 was approved in 2014 and released into the market in 2015, whereas the previous two were approved almost nine years prior (Durham et al. 2016). In a 2016 study, Gardasil-9 was determined to be the most cost-effective (Simms et al. 2016). From a biological standpoint, this makes sense; Gardasil-9 is so named because it protects against 9 different strains of HPV, while Gardasil and Ceravix protect against only 4 and 2, respectively. Researchers calculated the cost per quality-adjusted life year (QALY), or how much the vaccine would cost the patient for each year of health they gained, from a model using "a baseline scenario of vaccinating 10-year-old girls with 80% protection and 95% efficacy, at a cost of $95 per dose . . . and a 20 year duration" (Yi Yang and Bracken 2016). They found that the cost per QALY of Gardasil-9 was $12,208, which is more than $3,000 less than the cost per QALY of Gardasil (Yi Yang and Bracken 2016). The researchers maintained that as long as the price of Gardasil-9 did not surpass that of Gardasil by more than $11, this model would hold true. Another study performed by David P. Durham notes that to gain the same nationwide disease coverage from Gardasil and Ceravix combined, an additional 11 percent of the total population would need to be vaccinated, since they don't halt the spread of the disease as effectively. Over time, this would end up costing around "$2.7 billion more . . . than using [Gardasil-9] to achieve the same effect."

Now that it's been established which vaccine should be funded, it must be determined whether specific locations in the United States ought to receive the additional funding required for expanded distribution and administration of the vaccine, or whether funding should be given equally nationwide. Durham also conducted a study to answer this question in which three different scenarios were modeled and then compared: a 10 percent increase in national coverage of Gardasil-9 vaccination unilaterally, a 10 percent increase in coverage only in states that previously had low to no coverage, and a 10 percent increase in coverage only in states that previously had high coverage. The results were clear: increase in high-coverage states was projected to avert 9 cancers per 10,000 vaccines at the highest total cost, increase in national coverage was projected to avert 12 cancers per 10,000 vaccines at the median total cost, and increase in low-coverage states was projected to avert an impressive 20 cancers per 10,000 vaccines at the lowest total cost (Durham 2016). Durham also writes that "the effectiveness of expanded coverage in any one state is inversely proportional to the adolescent female coverage that has already been achieved in that state"; in other words, expanding coverage across the board and in states with high coverage is not nearly as effective as increasing funding in states with low coverage. So increasing coverage nationwide would not be the most effective use of funds; rather, a targeted approach should be used.

In conclusion, if we truly want to reduce the spread of HPV, funding must be poured into the Gardasil-9 vaccine, which is shown to be both the most protective and the most cost-effective, and vaccine coverage must be increased only in states that previously had low coverage. Not only will this save money, but it will also protect people from this dangerous virus.

References

Durham, David P., et al. 2016. "National- and State-Level Impact and Cost-Effectiveness of Nonavalent HPV Vaccination in the United States." *Proceedings of the National Academy of Sciences*, 113(18): 5107-5112. doi:10.1073/pnas.1515528113.

Simms, Kate T., et al. 2016. "Cost-effectiveness of the next Generation Nonavalent Human Papillomavirus Vaccine in the Context of Primary Human Papillomavirus Screening in Australia: a Comparative Modelling Analysis." *The Lancet Public Health*, 1(2): e66–e75. http://thelancet.com/journals/lanpub/article/PIIS2468-2667(16)30019-6/fulltext. Accessed on November 7, 2017.

Yi Yang, David, and Keyna Bracken. 2016. "Update on the New 9-Valent Vaccine for Human Papillomavirus Prevention." *Canadian Family Physician*, 62(5): 399–402.

Mia Tsang is a senior at Rhinebeck Senior High School in upstate New York who will be matriculating to Yale University. She plans to major in biology, but is also passionate about literature and writing.

HIV and Condom Negotiation
Liesl Nydegger

HIV among Young People

In the United States, HIV is primarily contracted via anal or vaginal sex, or sharing injection drug use equipment with a person who is HIV positive (Centers for Disease Control and Prevention [CDC] 2015). In 2015, almost a quarter of new HIV infections were among young people aged 13–24. Young people are at high risk for HIV due to inadequate sex education, the stigma around HIV, high rates of sexually transmitted infections (STIs), low rates of HIV testing, substance use, high number of sex partners, and low rates of condom use (CDC 2017).

HIV and Condoms

While abstinence is the only way to prevent HIV 100 percent, male and female condoms are highly effective in preventing HIV if used properly (CDC 2016a).

Table 3.1   Male Condom Dos and Don'ts

DO use a condom every time you have sex	DON'T store condoms in your wallet (heat/friction can damage them)
DO put on a condom before sex	DON'T use oil-based products (e.g., baby oil, lotion, petroleum jelly) as these will cause the condom to break
DO check the expiration date on the condom package	DON'T use more than one condom at a time
DO make sure there are no tears or defects in the condom	DON'T reuse a condom
DO use latex or polyurethane condoms	DON'T use lambskin condoms
DO use water-based or silicone-based lubricants	
DO store condoms in a cool, dry place	

Source: Centers for Disease Control and Prevention (2016b).

When using a male condom, you should (1) open the condom by tearing the wrapper on the side, (2) place the condom on the head of the erect penis, (3) pinch the air out of the tip of the condom, (4) unroll the condom all the way down to the base of the penis, (5) after sex but before pulling out, hold the condom at the base, then pull out while holding the condom in place, and (6) remove the condom and throw it in the trash (CDC 2016b).

When using a female condom, you should (1) open the condom by tearing the wrapper on the side, (2) squeeze the inner ring (the closed end) together and insert into vagina (similar to inserting a tampon), (3) use your finger and push the ring as far as it will go until it rests against your cervix and then the condom will expand naturally, (4) ensure the condom is not twisted and the thin outer ring should remain outside the vagina, (5) guide your partner's penis into the opening of the female condom, (6) remove the condom by gently twisting the outer ring and pull the female condom out, and (7) throw the female condom in the trash (CDC 2016c).

Condom Negotiation

Condom negotiation can be difficult, particularly for young people. It can be awkward if they are sexually inexperienced, if

Table 3.2   Female Condom Dos and Don'ts

DO use a female condom from start to finish (can be used for anal sex)	DON'T use a male condom with a female condom as this can cause tearing
DO read directions and check expiration date on the condom package	DON'T reuse a female condom
DO make sure there are no tears or defects in the condom	DON'T flush female condoms
DO use lubricant to prevent the condom from slipping or tearing	
DO store condoms in a cool, dry place	

Source: Centers for Disease Control and Prevention (2016c).

they are already inconsistent condom users, or if they mention HIV as HIV can be a stigmatized topic. There are six condom negotiation strategies that one can use: (1) *direct request* where one directly asks the partner to use a condom, (2) *withholding sex* where one refuses sex unless the partner agrees to use a condom, (3) *seduction* in which one partner gets the other one sexually aroused and then brings out a condom to use, (4) *relationship conceptualizing* where one expresses care and concern for the other person as a reason for wanting to use a condom, (5) *risk information* in which one person gives the other information about HIV and STIs to convince the other to use a condom, and (6) *deception* where one gives a deceptive reason for using a condom, such as pregnancy prevention when the true reason is HIV prevention (Holland and French 2012, 444).

It is common for young people to use more than one condom negotiation strategy, and those who use these strategies more often use condoms more frequently. Although men tend to use condoms more often than women, it is extremely important for women to become familiar and comfortable with these condom negotiation strategies in order to protect themselves from HIV and other STIs (Holland and French 2012, 450). Other studies among racial and ethnic minority young people found differing strategies preferred by different genders. For example, young Latino men used risk information and direct verbal/nonverbal communication whereas young Latinas tended to insist on condom use (Tschann et al. 2010, 259). Young African American women who were consistent condom users tended to withhold sex or use direct request strategies (McLaurin-Jones et al. 2016, 45). What is most important is that young people are aware of the different types of condom negotiation and are confident to use them in a sexual situation.

Conclusion

Young people are at risk for HIV and condoms are the most effective way of protection from HIV. They need to take the initiative to become their own advocate and protect themselves. Using these strategies will help, and role-playing with friends can help increase their confidence so when the time comes they are prepared.

References

Centers for Disease Control and Prevention. 2015. "HIV/AIDS: Risk by Age Group." www.cdc.gov/hiv/group/age/index.html. Accessed on May 15, 2017.

Centers for Disease Control and Prevention. 2016a. "HIV/AIDS: Prevention." www.cdc.gov/hiv/basics/prevention.html. Accessed on May 15, 2017.

Centers for Disease Control and Prevention. 2016b. "Male Condom Use." www.cdc.gov/condomeffectiveness/male-condom-use.html. Accessed on May 18, 2017.

Centers for Disease Control and Prevention. 2016c. "Female Condom Use." www.cdc.gov/condomeffectiveness/female-condom-use.html. Accessed on May 18, 2017.

Centers for Disease Control and Prevention. 2017. "HIV among Youth." www.cdc.gov/hiv/group/age/youth/index.html. Accessed on May 15, 2017.

Holland, Kathryn J., and Sabine E. French. 2012. "Condom Negotiation Strategy Use and Effectiveness among College Students." *Journal of Sex Research*, 49(5): 443–453.

McLaurin-Jones, Lashley TyWanda, Maudry-Beverly, and Vanessa Marshall. 2016. "Minority College Women's Views on Condom Negotiation." *International Journal of Environmental Research and Public Health*, 13(1): 40–51.

Tschann, Jeanne M., Elena Flores, Cynthia L. de Groat, Julianna Deardorff, and Charles J. Wibblesman. 2010. "Condom Negotiation Strategies and Actual Condom Use among Latino Youth." *Journal of Adolescent Health*, 47(3): 254–262.

Liesl Nydegger received her PhD and MPH from the School of Community and Global Health at Claremont Graduate University. Currently, she is an assistant professor in the Department of Kinesiology and Health Education at the University of Texas at Austin.

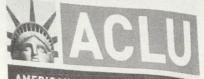

Introduction

The history of sexually transmitted infections (STIs) worldwide can sometimes best be understood and appreciated in the light of individuals who have spent their lives dealing with sexually transmitted diseases (STDs) and/or have made essential breakthroughs in our understanding of how those diseases are caused, the mechanisms by which they are transmitted, and the ways in which they can be prevented and treated. Many national and international organizations have made similar contributions, supporting essential research, providing aid and protection to those affected by the diseases, and helping to educate the general public about such diseases. This chapter provides brief sketches of some of the most important of those individuals and organizations.

Advocates for Youth

Advocates for Youth (AFY) was founded in 1980 to advocate for adolescent reproductive and sexual health. Its long history has been marked by a number of signal achievements, such as the following:

- Creation of the International Clearinghouse on Adolescent Fertility in 1980
- Production of a Life Planning Education program in 1983 that made sexuality a key element in the process of growing up

A member of Planned Parenthood speaks at a press conference about the organization's activities. (AP Photo/Rachel D'Oro)

- Establishment of the Support Center for School-Based Health Clinics in 1984 as a way of bringing health issues into the everyday life of adolescents in a school setting
- Sponsorship of a national AIDS (acquired immune deficiency syndrome) and adolescents conference in 1987 as one of the first efforts to deal with this rapidly growing and important issue in the area of adolescent sexual health
- Cosponsorship in 1992 of the first Inter-Africa Conference on Adolescent Reproductive Health
- Founder of the first online program for LGBT (lesbian, gay, bisexual, and transgender) youth, www.youthresource.com, and its Spanish-language sister site, www.ambientejoven.com

In addition to its expansive program on STIs, AFY conducts more than two dozen additional programs on topics such as abstinence, abortion, adolescent sexual health, condom efficacy and use, confidentiality in health care, contraceptive info and access, emergency contraception, LGBTQ (lesbian, gay, bisexual, transgender, and queer) issues, HIV, parent–child communication, policy and advocacy, sex education, violence and harassment, youth in low- and middle-income countries, and youth of color. A key element of the AFY effort is a K–12 curriculum that has been developed to deal with sexual issues for children and adolescents called Rights, Respect, and Responsibility. The program is available online at no charge to users at http://advocatesforyouth.org/3rs-curric-lessonplans.

Another important element of the organization's work is its policy and advocacy mission, through which it attempts to influence the views of state and federal legislators on topics of sexuality involving young adults. AFY has developed a number of resources to carry out this objective, including a Cultural Advocacy and Mobilization Initiative that works with individual states to help change uninformed and negative views about issues surrounding adolescent sexuality; a variety of policy publications, such as "Abstinence-Only-Until-Marriage Programs:

Ineffective, Unethical, and Poor Public Health," "Achieving the Millennium Development Goals," "Improving U.S. Global HIV Prevention for Youth," "Medical Organizations Support Condom Use," and "Youth in the Global Health Initiative."

Of special interest to professionals in the field of health education is a page on the organization's website providing a variety of resources that can be used in their work, such as a general introduction to the topic, Adolescent Sexual Health 101, examples of evidenced-based programs in sex education, training modules in adolescent sexual health, an overview of recommended school policies, suggestions for meeting the needs of youth at disproportionate risk, an introduction to the organization's SEA (state education agencies) annual institute, a list of resource of value to professionals in the field, and archives of the AFY School Health Equity newsletter. The website also provides links to six blogs addressing issues of special interest to adolescents: Youth Activists Bios (stories of individual adolescent sexual health advocates), Amplify (suggestions for youth who want to become active in AFY and related programs), Mysistahs (focusing on concerns of young women of color), Youthresource (written by and for LGBTQ youth), Ambiente Joven (a companion blog to Youthresource for Spanish-speaking youth), and Advocates' Youth Programs (designed to empower young leaders and activists). Another web page on the site is intended for parents, with a number of suggested resources for parents who want to learn more about and/or become more active in programs for improved education of and about adolescent sexual health.

American Sexual Health Association

The American Sexual Health Association (ASHA) was formed in New York City in 1914 as the result of the merger of two parent associations: the American Federation for Sex Hygiene, whose primary interest was the battle against STIs, and the American Vigilance Association, concerned primarily with the welfare of prostitutes. As has often been the case throughout history, issues of prostitution and STIs were closely associated, as they still are today. One of the organization's first campaigns involved the production of educational materials about STIs for military men fighting in World War I. The overarching message to these men was that members of the military had to be in prime health in order to carry out their assignments, and avoiding STIs was a crucial part of that task. At the same time, the ASHA was working to eliminate the primary source of this problem, the groups of prostitutes who gathered around military facilities and tended to promote the spread of STIs throughout the military. In 1914, the ASHA also began publishing two regular journals: *The Journal of Social Hygiene* and the *American Social Hygiene Association Bulletin*. The publications lasted until World War II, when they were both discontinued based on the success of penicillin in treating syphilis. Members of the association had come to believe that that success meant that syphilis would no longer be an issue of widespread concern in the United States and that the publications, therefore, were no longer needed.

The association no longer publishes a journal or newsletter, although it does carry and sell a wide array of publications on the topic of STIs. Some examples are books, booklets, and pamphlets, such as *Understanding Herpes, HPV and Cervical Cancer, Color Atlas and Synopsis of Sexually Transmitted Disease, HPV in Perspective, Syphilis and HIV: Make the Connection,* and *You Know about Syphilis, Right?* Among its most useful publications are a series of brochures on specific topics such as "What You Need to Know about HIV and AIDS," "What You Need to know about Gonorrhea," "Vaginitis," "Trichomoniasis," "Talking about Herpes," "Pelvic Inflammatory Disease," "Pap Tests: What Every Woman Should Know," and "NGU: A Man's Guide to a Common Sexually Transmitted Infection."

The association's website contains a page with very detailed and comprehensive information on virtually every aspect of STIs in which one would be interested, including an explanation of the difference between STDs and STIs, statistics on STIs, recommendations for ways in which one can reduce her or his risk for STIs, testing for STIs, methods of prevention, myths and facts, and descriptions of most STIs of interest, ranging from chlamydia, gonorrhea, and syphilis to molluscum, Mgen (*Mycoplasma genitalium*), and nongonococcal urethritis. Specific pages are also provided with information of particular interest to health providers, parents, and teachers.

American Sexually Transmitted Diseases Association

The American Sexually Transmitted Diseases Association (ASTDA) is an association whose members are interested and/or involved in research on STIs as well as efforts to control such diseases. Membership is open to any individual with such interests. The organization has three main functions: a biennial conference on STIs, publication of the journal *Sexually Transmitted Diseases*, and the presentations of three awards for distinguished contributions in the field—the ASTDA Achievement Award, the ASTDA Distinguished Career Award, and the Young Investigator Award. The Distinguished Career Award was originally given in 1972, and was named in honor of one of the great pioneers in the field of STIs and the sixth U.S. surgeon general, Thomas Parran. In 2013, the name of that award was changed to its current title because of new information about unethical research conducted in Guatemala by Parran between 1946 and 1948.

ASTDA can perhaps be regarded as the "granddaddy" of all U.S. organizations concerned with issues related to STIs. Its history dates back to 1934 and the founding of the American Neisserian Medical Society (ANMS). ANMS was itself the offshoot of an even early organization with the same objectives, the Neisserian Medical Society of Massachusetts. ANMS was concerned with a single disease, gonorrhea, focusing on methods for diagnosing, treating, and preventing the disease.

Within a few years, the attention and interest of the ANMS was drawn to a second STI, syphilis, largely as the result of efforts by Surgeon General Parran to draw the nation's attention to this newly important STI in the United States. During World War II, ANMS discontinued operations, and did not become active again until 1947. At that point, the medical community's attitudes about STIs had changed considerably, largely because of the success of penicillin in bringing gonorrhea and syphilis under control. The view at the time (later to be shown to be dramatically incorrect) was that both diseases, at least in the United States, had become issues of primarily historical interest. In response to this belief, ANMS changed its name in 1947 to the American Venereal Disease Association, reflecting a broader emphasis on all forms of STI. The association changed its name once more in 1976 to its present title.

In 1941, the organization took over management of a long-standing journal, *American Journal of Syphilis*, which had been founded in 1917, and renamed it the *American Journal of Syphilis, Gonorrhea, and Venereal Diseases*. (For a single issue, 1934–1935, the journal was called the *American Journal of Syphilis and Neurology*.) When the association broadened its sphere of interest to include other STIs, it also changed its name to the *American Journal of Syphilis, Gonorrhea, and Venereal Diseases*, and once more in 1974, to the *Journal of the American Venereal Disease Association*. Today, the journal is published under the name of *Sexually Transmitted Diseases*. It is published monthly and carries research on clinical, laboratory, immunologic, epidemiologic, behavioral, public health, and historical topics pertaining to STIs and related fields. It also carries reports from the Centers for Disease Control and Prevention (CDC) and National Institutes of Health (NIH) on the latest developments in the field of research.

amfAR: The Foundation for AIDS Research

The earliest stages of the AIDS epidemic in the 1980s met with considerable indifference and even ridicule. The disease was largely ignored by the medical profession as a whole, by policy makers and legislators, and by the general public. Underlying this lack of concern in many cases was the general feeling that those struck down by the disease somehow had called it upon themselves by adopting a dangerous and immoral lifestyle. Some religious leaders in particular felt that the disease was "God's punishment" for gay men's sins. One such leader, Jerry Falwell, went even a bit further when he said that "AIDS is not just God's punishment for homosexuals, it is God's punishment for the society that tolerates homosexuals."

The lack of public attention to the AIDS crisis was manifested to some extent by the decision by major health funding agencies to take up a program of research to learn more about the disease, its causes, and possible cures. To fill that gap, a handful of gay leaders and concerned nongays banded together in New York City in April 1983 to form the AIDS Medical Foundation (AMF). Probably the leading light in that effort was Dr. Mathilde Krim, then a researcher at Memorial Sloan Kettering Cancer Center in New York. The organization began an aggressive program of fund-raising and was able to make its first research grants less than a year of its creation. In September 1985, AMF combined forces with the National AIDS Research Foundation, which had been incorporated in California in August 1985. The new entity took the name of the Foundation for AIDS Research, known widely by its acronym of amfAR. In addition to its goal of collecting and distributing funds for research on the disease, amfAR also began an aggressive program of advertising about AIDS, providing accurate information on a disease that was otherwise surrounded by misunderstanding and fear.

Now, more than 30 years later, the organization has an impressive list of accomplishments to its credit. Of major importance has been the development of new drugs and new technologies for reducing the severity and limiting the spread of HIV infections. Although there is still no cure for HIV/AIDS, a very large fraction of individuals are now living long and productive lives because of the availability of these medications.

One of amfAR's current research priorities is the development of a vaccine against the disease.

amfAR has also supported other mechanisms for reducing the ravages of HIV/AIDS, perhaps most importantly syringe exchange programs that allow intravenous drug users to exchange used ("dirty") needles for safer clean needles. The organization has also provided financial support for studies that measure and evaluate the effectiveness of such programs.

Once progress was being made in the United States in the battle against AIDS, amfAR began to expand its work to other parts of the world. In 2001, as just one example, it founded TREAT Asia (Therapeutics Research, Education, and AIDS Training in Asia), a network of clinics, hospitals, and research institutions working with local, national, and regional governmental agencies, to ensure the safe and effective delivery of HIV/AIDS treatments throughout Asia and the Pacific. As of 2017, amfAR reports that the number of new infections in the region has fallen by about 20 percent, and the number of AIDS-related deaths by about 30 percent. During the same period, access to the retroviral treatment that can save people's lives has increased from 19 percent to 41 percent (as of 2015).

On a political level, amfAR has been involved in the development and adoption of a host of legislative initiatives designed to improve knowledge about, prevention of, and treatment for HIV infections. These initiatives have included federal legislation such as the Hope Act of 1988, the first federal legislation to address issues of HIV/AIDS; the Ryan White CARE Act of 1990, which provides emergency relief to states and local communities for a variety of HIV/AIDS services; the Americans with Disabilities Act of 1990, which adds people with AIDS to the list of those protected under the act; and the NIH Revitalization Act of 1993, which expanded the activities of the NIH's Office of AIDS.

In addition to TREAT Asia, amfAR has created a second international program, called the GMT Initiative. That program aids to provide research funds and technical support to workers in the field around the planet. The GMT acronym arises from the three major groups covered by the initiative: gay men, men who have sex with men (MSM), and transgender individuals.

According to its most recent annual report, the organization took in $46,610,198 during the fiscal year 2015, while disbursing $29,774,090 for research, public information, public policy activities, TREAT Asia, and the GMT Initiative.

Baruch S. Blumberg (1925–2011)

Blumberg was awarded a share of the 1976 Nobel Prize in physiology or medicine for his discovery of the virus that causes hepatitis B. That discovery made possible the development of a vaccine against the disease, an achievement for which Blumberg himself was largely responsible. Blumberg made this discovery, sometimes called one of the most important medical discoveries of the 20th century, quite by accident. At the time, he was engaged in an effort to discover why some ethnic groups appear to be more susceptible to some infectious diseases than are other ethnic groups. His attempts to resolve this puzzle involved taking blood samples from individuals from a great variety of ethnic groups throughout the world. One of his findings in this research had to do with a somewhat different question, the nature of a disease known at the time as serum hepatitis, or hepatitis B. Scientists had known for some time that two forms of hepatitis exist, one transmitted by the ingestion of contaminated foods, so-called infectious hepatitis, or hepatitis A, and serum hepatitis, or hepatitis B. Little was known about the cause of either disease.

In 1967, Blumberg discovered that individuals infected with hepatitis B in various parts of the world had antibodies in their blood for an antigen first discovered in the blood of Australian aborigines (and, therefore, called Australian antigen at the time). He eventually showed that this antigen consisted of a characteristic fragment of the outer shell of a virus, now known to be the virus that causes hepatitis B. With this information, Blumberg and his colleagues (in particular, American microbiologist Irving Millman) were able to design and produce a vaccine against the hepatitis B virus, which was licensed for use in the United States by the U.S. Food and Drug Administration (FDA) in 1969. More sophisticated vaccines have since been developed and approved by the FDA. Blumberg's discovery of the hepatitis B virus and his development of the corresponding vaccine are thought to have saved untold thousands of lives annually.

Baruch Samuel Blumberg was born in Brooklyn, New York, on July 28, 1925. He was the second of three children of Ida and Meyer Blumberg and the grandson of immigrants to the United States from Europe. He attended a yeshiva (Hebrew school) in Flatbush for his primary education and the Far Rockaway High School. He served in the U.S. Navy during World War II, which provided him with an opportunity to gain his college education under military sponsorship at Union College, in Schenectady, New York. Blumberg was graduated from Union in 1946 with his BS in physics. He then continued his studies in mathematics at Columbia University, but, at the suggestion of his father, switched to a medical program at the College of Physicians and Surgeons of Columbia in 1947. He received his MD from Columbia in 1951, and then remained at the Columbia Presbyterian Medical Center to complete his internship and residency. In 1955, Blumberg entered a doctoral program in biochemistry at Balliol College at Oxford University, in England, from which he received his PhD in 1957.

Blumberg's first professional assignment was at the NIH in Bethesda, Maryland, where he became involved in the formation and development of a new division on Geographic Medicine and Genetics. The mission of this division was to investigate the ways in which a person's or population's genetic makeup might affect their health and illness patterns, in general, and their susceptibility to infectious diseases, in particular. It was this background that eventually led Blumberg into the research that led to his discovery of the hepatitis B virus and vaccine.

In 1964, Blumberg was appointed associate director for clinical research at the Fox Chase Cancer Center in Philadelphia, a post he held until 1986. He also served at Fox Chase as distinguished scientist and senior advisor to the president. Beginning in 1964, Blumberg also had a long relationship with the University of Pennsylvania, where he was associate professor of medicine, human genetics, and anthropology (1964–1970), professor of medicine (1970–1977), professor of human genetics (1974–1977), professor of anthropology (1975–1977), and university professor of medicine and anthropology (1977–2011). He continued his connection with Balliol College, where he served as master from 1989 to 1994. In 1999, Blumberg's career took a somewhat different direction when he accepted the post of founding director of the Astrobiology Institute of the National Aeronautics and Space Administration (NASA) at the Ames Research Center in Moffet Field, California. He was also senior advisor to the NASA administrator in Washington, D.C., from 2000 to 2001. After leaving the Astrobiology Institute, Blumberg continued his affiliation with NASA by taking a post as distinguished scientist at the NASA Lunar Science Institute at Ames Research Center.

Blumberg's special expertise in the field of medical anthropology has made him in demand at universities and research centers around the world. He has been visiting professor or researcher at the University of Kentucky, Indiana University, Stanford University, University of Washington, University of Otago (New Zealand), Trinity College of Oxford University, University of Bangalore, University of Singapore, and the Stazione Zoologica Anton Dohrn of Naples. In addition to the Nobel Prize, he has been awarded the Passano Award, the Karl Landsteiner Memorial Award, the Richard & Hinda Rosenthal Foundation Award, the Molly & Sidney Zubrow Award, the Sammy Davis Junior National Liver Institute Award, the Showa Emperor (Japan) Memorial Award, and the Gold Medal

Award of the Canadian Liver Foundation and Canadian Association for the Study of the Liver.

Blumberg died of a heart attack on April 5, 2011, shortly after giving the keynote speech at the International Lunar Research Park Exploratory Workshop being held at the Ames Research Center.

John C. Cutler (1915–2003)

In an obituary on the occasion of his death, Cutler was described as a leader in "trying to prevent and control sexually transmitted diseases around the world." He was widely admired and respected as a teacher, researcher, and administrator of programs for the control and treatment of STIs. During World War II, Cutler was actively involved in efforts to understand and implement the use of penicillin in the treatment of syphilis and gonorrhea among U.S. military forces. Cutler is also remembered as director of a series of experiments in which uninformed individuals in a handful of developing nations were used as "guinea pigs," without their consent, to study the characteristic features and methods of treating syphilis and gonorrhea.

John Charles Cutler was born on June 29, 1915, to Glen Allen and Grace Amanda Allen Cutler. He attended primary and secondary schools in Cleveland before matriculating at Western Reserve University (now Case Western University), from which he graduated in 1941. A year later, he accepted an appointment the U.S. Public Health Service (PHS), where he served as a medical officer at the agency's Venereal Disease Research Laboratory on Staten Island, New York. He later became involved in a series of experiments on methods for treating syphilis that began with a project in Guatemala in 1946. In that project, an estimated 1,500 prisoners, military personnel, orphans, prostitutes, and other men and women were inoculated with the causative agents for syphilis, gonorrhea, and chancroid. The goal of the experiment was to determine the effect of penicillin as a treatment for the diseases among American military personnel returning to the United States after the end of World War II. (For more details on this event, see Rory Carroll, "Guatemala Victims of US Syphilis Study Still Haunted by the 'Devil's Experiment,'" *The Guardian*, https://www.theguardian.com/world/2011/jun/08/guatemala-victims-us-syphilis-study, accessed on March 25, 2017.)

Cutler was also involved in what is probably the most notorious research study in the history of U.S. medicine, the Tuskegee (Alabama) syphilis study. That project, which ran from 1932 to 1972, was designed to learn more about the stages of development of syphilis in otherwise healthy (and exclusively black) men in Alabama. As with the Guatemala studies, subjects were inoculated with *Treponema pallidum*, without their informed consent. The experiment was continued long after medical authorities were aware that the disease could be cured or controlled by the administration of penicillin. As a consequence, many of those subjects eventually developed third-stage syphilis, from which they experienced debilitating consequences and even death.

In a somewhat less controversial experiment, Cutler was also in charge of a study at New York state's Sing Sing prison beginning in 1954. In this case, prisoners were inoculated with the killed *T. pallidum* bacterium to see if it would prevent development of the disease. In this case, however, subjects were eventually treated, and usually cured, of the syphilis that developed as a result of the experiment.

In 1958, Cutler was promoted to assistant surgeon general of the United States, a post he held for less than two years. He then accepted an appointment with the Allegheny County Health Department, where he was in charge of the local polio vaccination program. A year later, in 1961, he returned to Washington, where he served first as assistant, and later as deputy director, of the Pan American Sanitary Organization, forerunner of today's Pan American Health Organization (PAHO). In 1967, he left PAHO to become professor of international health and head of the population division in the Graduate School of Public Health at the University of Pittsburgh. He later served also as chairman of the university's Department of Health Administration and dean of the graduate school in 1968 and 1969. He remained at Pittsburgh until his retirement in 1985. Cutler died in Pittsburgh on February 8, 2003, at the age of 87. In 2011, Wellesley College researcher Susan M. Reverby published a paper on her review of Cutler's role in the Guatemala and Tuskegee experiments, a role that was at the time not well known. In response to this news, the University of Pittsburgh discontinued an annual lecture series created in his honor following Cutler's death.

Division of STD Prevention

The Division of STD Prevention (DSTDP) is a section within the CDC's National Center for HIV/AIDS, Viral Hepatitis, STD and TB Prevention (NCHHSTP). Its primary mission is to help individuals reduce their risk of STIs and the transmission of those diseases throughout society. In order to achieve this objective, DSTDP sponsors and conducts a wide range of activities and events for policy makers, parents, young adults, and others interested in issues related to STIs. An important tool of the agencies work is the grants it is able to provide for research, training, and education on STI issues throughout the country. As of 2017, DSTDP was supporting STI prevention programs in all 50 states, 7 cities (Los Angeles, San Francisco, the District of Columbia, Chicago, Baltimore, New York City, and Philadelphia), and 2 territories (Puerto Rico and the U.S. Virgin Islands).

DSTDP takes a multifaceted approach to dealing with STIs at the local, state, and federal levels. An example of a program that has now been completed is the Infertility Prevention Project, cosponsored with the Office of Population Affairs of the Department of Health and Human Services. The purpose of that project was to provide funding for low-income, sexually active women to have access to screening and treatment programs for gonorrhea and chlamydia. Both of these diseases can have long-term effects on a woman's reproductive system. By reducing the rate of the two diseases among the target population, then, can be an important step in reducing the infertility rate among women of childbearing age.

Another example of a DSTDP program has been the Community Approaches to Reducing Sexually Transmitted Diseases initiative, which ran from September 2014 to September 2017. This program was aimed specifically at reducing the disparities for STIs among various subgroups within the population, such as people of color and LGBTQ youth. As part of this project, DSTDP funded local projects at the Chicago AIDS Foundation of Chicago, Baltimore City Health Department, Public Health Management Corporation of Philadelphia, and the University of Michigan. An important ongoing activity of the department is the STD Surveillance Network. An important objective of this program is improving the methods for collecting data about STIs to provide researchers, administrators, and clinicians with reliable information about the behavioral, demographic, and clinic aspects of various STIs as an efficient way of improving prevention and treatment options to specific agencies. One product of this line of research is the annual *Sexually Transmitted Disease Surveillance*, which summarizes data provided by dozens of local and state STI agencies as to the number of STI cases annually in the United States, as well as demographic correlates within the data, such as sex, age, racial and ethnic background, and geographical location.

Improving the knowledge and skills of workers in the field is another aspect of the DSTDP agenda. Among the resources provided by the department are a collection of courses on clinical, behavioral, and public health aspects of STIs; continuing online education courses; comprehensive curriculum materials for sex educators on seven specific STIs; a self-directed and STI-focused SAS (a computer program) training module; "STD in a Box," a collection of materials that can be used for individualized STI prevention workshops; STD clinical slides, a presentation that describes the symptoms of various STIs; and STD picture cards that provides illustrated information comparable to that available in STD clinical slides.

The organization's website also provides a wealth information on specific STIs, along with additional discussions of STI-related issues, such as STIs and infertility, STIs during pregnancy, risks for STIs associated with oral sex, and information on some STIs that are perhaps less well known and less frequently discussed, such as chancroid, lymphogranuloma venereum, pubic lice, and scabies.

Paul Ehrlich (1854–1915)

Ehrlich was a German bacteriologist who was awarded a share of the 1908 Nobel Prize in physiology or medicine for his research on autoimmunity, the process by which a body develops immune responses against its own tissues, cells, or other components. In the area of sexual health, he is best known for his discovery of the first safe and effective treatment for syphilis, one of the most terrible diseases in human history.

Paul Ehrlich was born on March 14, 1854, in Strehlen, Silesia, then a part of Prussia, a city now known as Strzelin, in modern Poland. He completed his secondary education at the Breslau Gymnasium (high school), and then studied medicine at the universities of Breslau, Strasbourg, Freiburg, and Leipzig, from which he received his medical degree in 1877. His doctoral dissertation dealt with the staining of cells, a topic that was to remain a centerpiece of his research for the rest of his life. In 1878, Ehrlich accepted an appointment as a researcher at the Berlin Medical Clinic, where he later had an opportunity to work with the famous Robert Koch on the tubercle bacillus responsible for tuberculosis. During this research, Ehrlich caught a mild case of the disease and traveled to Egypt for two years in order to live and work in a more amenable climate. Some biographers have surmised that this experience was a seminal factor in developing Ehrlich's overall view to the search for methods of treating disease. He envisioned finding a "magic bullet," some compound that would attack disease-causing microorganisms only, without affecting beneficial organisms or an animal's body. His work on staining suggested that some compound must exist, compounds that recognize and attach themselves only to specific microorganisms. His goal was to find compounds that were effective in bonding to bacteria and other disease-causing microorganisms and then attach to the stain a poison that would kill the organism.

Over the years, Ehrlich methodically worked his way through hundreds of potential stains that might be used as a "magic bullet." In 1909, one of his assistants, Sachahiro Hata, returned to a compound that had already been tested and rejected, called compound 606 because it was the 606th compound to have been tested. (At this point, Ehrlich was already working on compounds 900+.) Hata found that the compound was very effective in killing the spirochete that causes syphilis, *T. pallidum*. In 1910, the compound was made generally available to physicians under the name of salvarsan. It, along with a related drug called neosalvarsan, were the only safe and effective drugs for the treatment of syphilis until penicillin became generally available for this purpose in the 1940s.

Ian Frazer (1953–)

Frazer invented a vaccine against the human papillomavirus (HPV), which is the causative agent in the vast majority of cervical cancer, the third most common type of cancer among women worldwide. The virus has also been implicated in a number of other types of cancers of the genital system, including vaginal, vulvar, uterine, and ovarian cancers, as well as anal cancer in men. HPV is also the most common STI, responsible for genital warts and other types of oral and genital infections. The invention of a vaccine to prevent the transmission of HPV holds the promise for saving millions of lives annually world-wide from cervical and other types of cancer.

Ian Hector Frazer was born in Glasgow, Scotland, on January 6, 1953. At the age of three, he moved with his family to Edinburgh, where his father took a position in biochemistry at Edinburgh University, while his mother continued her career as a medical researcher. With that type of background, it is hardly surprising that young Ian soon became interested in science. In a 2006 interview with Australian television channel ABC1, Frazer noted that he was "really fascinated by how things worked, what made them happen, why they didn't always happen, and that became a driving force in what I actually did at school." He attended George Watson's College, a private primary and secondary school in Edinburgh, before enrolling at the University of Edinburgh. Torn between a career in physics and a career in medicine, he finally chose the latter because he thought it provided more research opportunities. He eventually earned his bachelor of science degree in pathology in 1974 and his bachelor of medicine and bachelor of surgery in 1977, both from Edinburgh. He completed his residencies at Edinburgh Eastern General Hospital, the Edinburgh Royal Infirmary, and the Roodlands General Hospital in Haddington, Scotland.

In 1981, Frazer emigrated to Australia to take a position as senior research officer at the Walter and Eliza Hall Institute in Melbourne. He left the Hall Institute in 1985 to become director of the Division of Clinical Immunology at the Princess Alexandra Hospital in Brisbane, a post he held until 1999. Between 1989 and 1993, Frazer also served simultaneously as associate professor in the Department of Medicine at the University of Queensland. In 1994, he was promoted to full professor at the University of Queensland. In 1991, Frazer also accepted an appointment as director of the Center for Immunology and Cancer Research (now the Diamantina Institute) at the University of Queensland, a post he continues to hold. In 1994, he added the title of professor in the Department of Medicine at the university.

Frazer's interest in an HPV vaccine dates to the late 1980s when he first discussed the problems of developing such a vaccine with Chinese virologist Jian Zhou. The basic problem the two researchers faced was a classic challenge for inventors of a vaccine: to develop a product that will convince the human immune system of the presence of a harmful substance (the HPV) without actually using material sufficiently virulent to induce the disease itself. The problem was eventually resolved by Jian's wife, Xiao-Yi Sun, who used the methods of recombinant DNA to produce a synthetic particle that closely resembled the shell of the HPV. That resemblance was sufficiently close that, when injected into a human, the synthetic particle produced essentially the same immune response as did the HPV itself. After more than five years of testing, the synthetic vaccine was approved for human use in the United States by the FDA in 2006. It is now available in two proprietary formulations known as Gardasil® and Cervaris®.

(Although sometimes given lesser attention, Jian's contribution to the development of the vaccine was substantial. In fact, he is often referred to as an "equal partner" in the project. Jian's life was tragically cut short in 1999 when, at the age of 42, he died as the result of complications arising out of a routine medical procedure in Australia. An important memorial to Jian and his work is available at http://www.scribd.com/doc/2740521/zhou-jianprefaces-Etc.)

In the years following licensing of the HPV vaccine, Frazer has received a number of awards and honors including the Howard Florey Medal for Medical Research, Prime Minister's Prize for Science, Balzan Prize for Preventive Medicine, Australian Medical Association Gold Medal, William B. Cooley Award, CSIRO Eureka Prize for Leadership in Science, Centenary Medal for services to cancer research, Ramaciotti Medal, American Academy of Dermatology Lila Gruber Award for Dermatology, Novartis Prize for Clinical Immunology, Golden Plate Award of the International Achievement Summit, International Life Award for Scientific Research, Merck Sharp &

Dohme Howard Florey Medal, Clunies Ross Award of the Academy of Technological Sciences and Engineering, Distinguished Fellowship Award of the Royal College of Pathologists, and John Curtin Medal. In 2006, he was named Australian of the Year and Queenslander of the Year, and in 2012, he was named a National Living Treasure by the National Trust of Australia.

Gay Men's Health Crisis

The fall of 1981 was rapidly becoming a terrifying period for the gay community of the United States. Reports were coming in about a type of "gay cancer" that had never before been seen among healthy young men. By the end of that year, 121 men had died of the disease, a number that rose to 447 a year later, and to 1,476 in 1983. As rapidly as the disease spread through the gay community, so did the realization among many gay men and lesbians that help from federal and nongovernmental agencies for help in dealing with the epidemic was likely not to be quickly forthcoming. A number of individuals in position of responsibility proclaimed that AIDS (the "gay cancer") was retribution from God for the immoral lifestyles of those affected. And with public approval of homosexual behavior at a very low level in the country, there was little general outcry for efforts to combat the disease.

As it happened, however, a relatively small group of gay men and their supporters recognized the medical challenge of dealing with this new STI very early on in the epidemic. One such group met on August 11, 1981, in New York City, to form an organization to begin dealing with the disease. The group collected $7,000 from its members and created the Gay Men's Health Crisis (GMHC), an organization that continues to serve HIV/AIDS patients and at-risk populations today.

GMHC has an extensive variety of programs designed to help people learn their HIV status and to find ways of dealing with those who are positive. Some of the many services include the following:

- Confidential HIV testing is provided to anyone wishing the service at no charge through the David Geffen Center for HIV Prevention and Health Education.

- Anyone who tests positive for HIV is directed to a variety of local community health resources that can assist them with their medical, social, emotional, financial, and other HIV-related issues.

- The Community Health and Research services at the GMHC Center for HIV Prevention works with individuals at high risk for HIV, especially youth, women, and people of color, to provide educational opportunities, counseling, social events, and other activities.

- Legal, Client Advocacy and Client Financial Services assist HIV-positive individuals with services designed to help them deal with the challenges of everyday life as a result of the disease, such as avoiding eviction from their places of lodging; gaining access to benefits; pursuing claims of discrimination; applying for legal documents such as passports and green cards; and helping with social security, Medicare, Medicaid, and related issues.

- Mental health services are provided by GMHC through its Michael Palm Center for AIDS Care and Support. These services include individual and group counseling that are available to anyone interested in participating, including HIV-positive individuals, those at risk for the disease, and MSM.

- The organization's Action Center provides a venue through which interested individuals can meet and discuss issues of public policy related to HIV/AIDS.

- The Expanded Syringe Access Program runs a needle exchange program.

- Nutrition counseling and education are provided through both individual counseling and group programs.

In a review of the center's most recent accomplishment, current director Kelsey Louie noted the center's most notable accomplishments for 2016: service to more than 10,000 clients in New York City that included more than 3,000 HIV tests, complemented by a 90 percent viral suppression rate among those who test positive. During the period, GMHC also provided more than 80,000 hot meals to people living with AIDS, as well as opening a new center devoted specifically to the needs of youth.

Ludwig Halberstädter (1876–1949)

Halberstädter, along with Czech zoologist Stanislaus von Prowazek, is credited with the discovery of the bacterium *Chlamydia trachomatis* in 1907. Four years earlier, von Prowazek and Halberstädter had traveled with Polish physician and researcher Albert Neisser to the island of Java in the Dutch East Indies (now Indonesia) in a search for the causative agent of syphilis. During the expedition, von Prowazek and Halberstädter also conducted a series of experiments attempting to discover the causative agent of trachoma, a common bacterial infection of the eye that can lead to blindness. As part of the experiments, they transplanted material from the eyes of individuals with trachoma to the eyes of orangutans, the species that share many biological characteristics of humans. Upon taking scrapings from the orangutan eyes, they discovered new types of structures, later known as Halberstädter-Prowazek bodies, or Halberstädter-Prowazek inclusions that contained a new type of bacterium, now known by the name of *C. trachomatis*. The discovery was the single most important accomplishment in Halberstädter's long research career.

Ludwig Halberstädter was born on December 9, 1876, in Beuthen, Oberschlesien, Germany. He attended Breslau

University (now the University of Wroclaw in Poland), from which he received his doctoral degree in radiology in 1901. Following his graduation, he took a post in the surgical clinic at the University of Königsberg, where he served until 1907. He then returned to Breslau, where he worked as an assistant to Neisser in the dermatology clinic. It was during this period that he became involved in Neisser's own research and traveled with him (and von Prowazek) to Java.

After the East Indies expedition, Halberstädter returned to Breslau where he specialized in the study of the effects of radiation on dermatological conditions. In 1919, he was made head of the department of radiology at the University of Berlin, after which he was also named lecturer (1921) and then professor (1926) at Berlin. In 1933, as part of the new National Socialist (Nazi) government actions, and along with thousands of his Jewish academic colleagues, Halberstädter was dismissed from his post in Berlin, but allowed to leave the country. He traveled to Palestine, where he became head of the radiology department at Hadassah Hospital in Jerusalem, where he continued his research and teaching for more than a decade. He died in New York City on August 20, 1949, while on a visit to the United States, a few months before he was to retire from his post in Jerusalem. In an academic career that stretched over four decades, he published more than a hundred peer-reviewed papers and became a favorite teacher among his many students.

Hippocrates (ca. 460 BCE to ca. 370 BCE)

Hippocrates is generally regarded as the most famous physician in the ancient world, and one of the greatest figures ever in the history of medicine. He described a disease that he called *stangury*, that was probably gonorrhea, and another condition that was almost certainly a type of hepatitis. In addition to the description of a number of other medical conditions, Hippocrates is remembered for a general framework of the medical sciences, much of which remains as part of medical practice.

For example, he described various categories of illness, including epidemics and endemic events, as well as pointing out the differences between acute and chronic forms of an illness. He is perhaps best known to the general public for the Hippocratic Oath, which, traditionally, all physicians take when they have completed their medical training. The nine parts of the oath include a promise to acknowledge when one does not know the answer to a question, to respect the privacy of patients, to prevent disease wherever possible, and to remember that he or she is a member of society with certain special obligations to his or her fellow man or woman. Perhaps the requirement most often associated with the oath, "First, I will do no harm," was not actually a part of the original statement, although that prescription is clearly part of Hippocrates's other writings.

Very little is known with certainty about the life of Hippocrates. We know something of his fame as a physician from the writings of two contemporaries, Plato and Meno, Hippocrates's student. Plato referred to Hippocrates as "the asclepiad (physician) of Cos" and briefly described his philosophy of medicine. Meno also discussed Hippocrates's medical views and illustrated how they differed from the prevailing wisdom of the type. The vast majority of works that are attributed to his name are probably the works of other authors. His reputation was so great for such a long period of time that medical writers thought it judicious to place his name on their own works, thus making it difficult, if not impossible, to know precisely what he thought, practiced, and wrote. There is no doubt, however, of his enormous influence on the medical profession for a thousand years or more after his death.

Hippocrates is thought to have been born on the Greek island of Cos (Kos), and died in the town of Larissa about 60 years later. His first biographer was Soranus, a physician from Ephesus who wrote about Hippocrates about 500 years after his death, leaving in doubt even the most basic information about the physician's life.

International Society for Sexually Transmitted Diseases Research

The purpose of the International Society for Sexually Transmitted Diseases Research is to promote research on STIs. The organization's primary activity is a biennial conference on STIs, held alternately in Europe and North America. Among the topics discussed at these meetings are HIV infections and the AIDS; microbiology; virology; immunobiology; pathogenesis; clinical sciences; social and behavioral sciences; epidemiology; prevention; and research in health services, public health, and prevention policy.

International Union against Sexually Transmitted Infections

The International Union against Sexually Transmitted Infections (IUSTI) was founded in 1923 and claims to be the oldest international organization working to foster international cooperation in controlling the spread of STIs. Membership in IUSTI is open to individuals on a full or associate basis and to organizations and commercial sponsors. The organization sponsors annual international conferences, as well as regional and international conferences and other meetings, on specific topics such as HIV/AIDS, the HPV, neisseria vaccines, and clinical microbiology and infectious diseases. It carries out much of its work through five regional affiliates in Africa, Asia Pacific, Europe, Latin America, and North America. The association publishes two journals: the *International Journal of STD & AIDS* and *Sexual Health—The Official Journal of IUSTI—Asia-Pacific*.

Larry Kramer (1935–)

Larry Kramer is a playwright and screenwriter who had been active in the campaign against HIV for more than three decades. It is manifestly impossible to feature in this chapter any one individual among the countless number of workers who organized and fought against the HIV epidemic from the early 1980s onward. And Kramer is clearly one of the most controversial of those individuals, as much among his fellow gay men and lesbian colleagues as among the general public. However, very few, if any, individuals have made a more significant contribution to the gay and lesbian community's efforts to understand HIV and to organize to help the community survive the epidemic than Kramer.

Laurence David Kramer was born on June 25, 1935, in Bridgeport, Connecticut, to George L. and Rea Wishengard Kramer. Although he had earned a law degree from Yale, the elder Kramer had a falling out with his brother in New York City, and the family moved to Bridgeport, where they took up occupancy in a third-floor apartment above a grocery store owned by his maternal grandparents. In Depression times, George Kramer was unsuccessful in finding work, and as Larry Kramer later noted, he "never made a dime from 1931 to 1939," and his mother worked to support the family.

Kramer entered Yale University in 1953, where he did quite poorly and suffered from periods of depression because of his feelings for other men. As did many gay men of the time, he felt then that he was the only person in the world with such feelings and attempted suicide during his freshman year. He eventually gravitated toward the theater department at Yale, where he felt comfortable for the first time. He also began psychoanalytical counseling, which he later praised for having "saved his life."

After earning a bachelor's degree from Yale in English in 1957, Kramer served briefly in the U.S. Army Reserves before finding a position as a mail clerk at the William Morris Agency in New York City. The agency was a talent agency that has for many decades represented some of the most famous entertainment figures in the United States and elsewhere. After a short period of time with William Morris, Kramer left the company to take a job as teletype operator at Columbia Pictures. He stayed at Columbia for only a year before joining the Neighborhood Playhouse to study acting. That experience was also a brief interlude, and he returned to Columbia in 1960, where he worked as a script reader. In 1961, he was asked by Columbia to move to London to direct a story department for the company. While there, Kramer was involved in the production of a number of major motion pictures, including *Lawrence of Arabia*, *Dr. Strangelove*, and *Women in Love*, for which he won an Oscar nomination for screenplay.

By 1972, Kramer had left London, with some regrets, to return to New York, where he began working on a number of projects, including a play about four friends from Yale, three heterosexuals and one homosexual. The play was unsuccessful and Kramer next turned his attention to narrative fiction, producing his first major novel in 1978, *Faggots*. That career was put on hold with the arrival of the AIDS epidemic, into which he threw all of his energies for a number of years. The story of his involvement during that period is long and complex. He took the position that only a radical change in lifestyles by gay men, such as discontinuing multiple sexual contacts and avoiding gay bathhouses, could bring the epidemic under control. He made his views clear forcefully, often in terms that offended his closest allies in the battle. He was even forcibly removed from leadership positions at GMHC by colleagues who could no longer tolerate his abusive manner. In 1987, Kramer was also one of the founding members of an organization called ACT UP (AIDS Coalition to Unleash Power) designed to provide services to HIV-positive individuals and members of at-risk groups, such as MSM and injection drug users.

Kramer later told the story of this period and the travails of his interactions with others in the Broadway play "The Normal Heart." The play was later made into a 2014 television film, starring Mark Ruffalo, that won a number of honors, including Best Miniseries from the Golden Globe Awards, Best Movie from the Critics' Choice Television Awards, Outstanding Television Movie from the Primetime Emmy Awards, and the Stanley Kramer Award of the Producers Guild of America Awards.

At the age of 82, Kramer continues to be active in speaking and writing about important issues in modern life, most commonly HIV disease and people who have been and are affected by it. In 1993, he was named a Pulitzer Prize finalist for his play, *The Destiny of Me*, and, in 2013, he was given a Master American Dramatist award by the PEN/Laura Pels International Foundation for Theater Awards

Luc Montagnier (1932–)

Montagnier was awarded a share of the 2008 Nobel Prize in physiology or medicine for his part in the discovery of the virus that causes HIV/AIDS disease. That award was surrounded by a considerable amount of controversy because it did not also include a person sometimes thought to be a codiscoverer, American biomedical researcher, Robert Gallo.

In the early 1980s, the sudden appearance and rise of AIDS cases in the United States and other parts of the world prompted researchers in a number of countries to begin looking for a possible causative agent. In early 1983, Montagnier and his colleagues discovered a candidate for this role, a virus they called LAV (lymphadenopathy-associated virus). Much of the actual research involved in this accomplishment was conducted by and under the direction of French virologist Francoise Barré-Sinoussi, who worked under Montagnier's direction at Pasteur Institute at Paris and who won a share of the 2008 Nobel Prize with Montagnier.

In July 1983, Montagnier's team provided samples of the LAV to laboratories around the world working on the problem who had requested them. One such individual was Gallo, then working at the National Cancer Institute. Although Gallo and his team continued work on the LAV, they eventually came to the conclusion that another causative agent was involved, a virus they named human T-cell lymphotropic virus

III (HTLV-III), the third of a group of disease-causing organisms that they had discovered. In early 1984, the Gallo team published a series of papers suggesting that HTLV-III was the causative agent for HIV.

A long controversy followed as to which research team, the French or American, was correct, and which should receive credit for discovery of the HIV. The debate became so contentious that legal issues eventually arose to tarnish the reputation of both teams. To some extent, but not to everyone's satisfaction, the issue was eventually laid to rest with the award of the Nobel Prize in 2008 to Montagnier and Barré-Sinoussi (an award they also shared with Harald zur Hausen for his research on the viral origin of diseases).

Luc Montagnier was born on August 18, 1932, in Chabris, France, a community he later described as "larger than a village, but smaller than a town." The first 10 years of his life were marked by the horrors of World War II, a time during which his own home was partially demolished by a bomb from the Allied forces' air force. He attended local primary and secondary schools where, as he later said, was "usually ahead of his classmates." As with many scientific leaders, he felt the pull of science and technology early in his life, fascinated by electric batteries and the products that he could make with a home chemistry set.

Upon graduation from the Collège de Châtellerault, Montagnier decided to continue his studies at both the Faculty of Sciences and the School of Medicine in Poitiers. His plan was to start on a career in research on human biology, and this plan allowed him to attend classes at one facility in the morning, and then walk to classes in the other facility in the afternoon. He received the French equivalent of a bachelor's degree in natural sciences in 1953. He then went on to earn his licentiate in science and his medical degree from the University of Paris in 1955 and 1960 respectively.

Upon completing his studies, Montagnier accepted an offer to complete his postdoctoral studies at the Medical Research

Council at Carshalton in the United Kingdom. Three years later, he moved to the Institute of Virology, in Edinburgh, Scotland. It was at Carshalton and Edinburgh that he made some of his most important discoveries about the nature and reproduction of viruses in a variety of settings. In 1965, he returned to France, where he continued his research on viruses as laboratory director of the Institut du Radium (later, the Institut Curie). Seven years later, he moved again, this time to the Institut Pasteur in Paris, where he founded and became director of the Viral Oncology Unit at the Virology Department of the Pasteur Institut.

Over the next three decades, Montagnier held a variety of research and administration posts, often simultaneously, in the field of virology. These included director of research at the CNRS (Le Centre national de la recherche scientifique), one of the most prestigious scientific institutions in Europe (and the world), 1974–1998; chief of the virology department and head of the postgraduate course on general virology at the Pasteur Institut, 1980–1985; professor at the Pasteur Institut, 1985–2000; chief of the retrovirus department at the Pasteur, 1991–1997; and distinguished professor and director of the Center of Molecular and Cellular Biology at Queens College, New York. He officially retired from active research and was named director of research emeritus at CERN (Conseil Européen pour la Recherche Nucléaire; European Council for Nuclear Research; 1999) and professor emeritus at the Pasteur (2000). In 1993, Montagnier was also named president of the UNESCO's World Foundation for AIDS Research and Prevention.

In 2010, Montagnier provided evidence that his research career was not yet over, even at the age of 78, when he accepted an appointment at the Shanghai Jiao Tong University (SJTU). He was to continue his research in a building especially provided for him in the School of Life Sciences and Biology at the Minhang campus of SJTU. He was also to serve as director of a new institute, the Montagnier Institute, created in his honor.

Montagnier's work has been recognized with a long list of honors and awards, including Knight of the Legion of Honour, Commander of the National Order of Merit, Officer of the Legion of Honour, Commander of the Legion of Honour, Officer of the Mayo Order (Argentina), Grand Officer of the Legion of Honour, Rozen prize for cancerology, bronze and silver medal of the CNRS, Gallien prize, Louis Jeantet prize, James Blundel prize, Korber Foundation for European Research prize, Albert Lasker prize, Gairdner prize, Japan prize, King Faisal Prince of Saudi Arabia International prize for medicine, Amsterdam Foundation for Medicine prize of the Dutch Royal Academy of Sciences, Atomic Energy Committee prize, Hippocrates prize of the Hellenic Society for Internal Medicine, Neil Hamilton Fairley prize of the Royal College of Physicians of London, Steve Chase humanitarian prize, Rome Frégéné prize, Japanese Red Cross prize, German Red Cross prize, Warren Alpert prize, Recherche et Médecine prize of the Institut des Sciences de la Santé (Paris), Prince of Asturias Award, Laureate of the National Inventors Hall of Fame, Prestige EDC Prize of Ecole des Dirigeants et Créateurs d'entreprises (Paris), Prize of the Académie des sciences médicales of Bilbao, and the prize of the MBC News of Dubaï. He has also been awarded honorary doctorates at more than a dozen major universities, including the universities of Leuven, Liege, Salonica, Albert Einstein College of Medicine, American University of Paris, Bologna, Buenos Aires, Urbino (Italy), Montreal, Laval, London, Bucharest, and Athens.

National Coalition of STD Directors

The National Coalition of STD Directors (NCSD) was incorporated in 1997 for the purpose of working for the development of national policies and practices that promote sexual health and public awareness of important issues associated with STDs. NCSD consists of 65 federally funded programs, 50 at the state level, 8 at the city level, and 7 located in territories.

The organization is under the control of a board of directors consisting of individual directors of member organizations and operated by a Washington D.C.-based staff currently led by executive director David C. Harvey. The organization's six major objectives are to

- create a full partnership among STD project areas directly funded by the CDC, state and local public health agencies, the federal government, and private agencies to effectively prevent and control STDs in the United States and its territories;
- provide a conduit of communication and technology transfer among and between STD directors nationally;
- provide a forum for technical assistance and dissemination of information about effective STD prevention and control programs among members of the coalition;
- educate federal, state, and local policy makers about issues relevant to STD control and prevention;
- network or affiliate with appropriate organizations working toward comparable goals;
- promote adequate and efficient allocation of resources to STD sexual health promotion.

One prong of the organization's efforts is to better educate the general public and policy makers about the nature of STDs, their current status in the United States, research in the field, and desirable policies and programs. To carry out this function, NCSD issues a variety of print and electronic materials, including press releases, policy statements, policy updates, and news articles about STDs. Examples of such publications are a 2010 policy statement on worker health and safety and the adult film industry, a number of policies statements on STD issues arising out of the new administration of President Donald Trump, and a news report on the organization's release of a half million condoms to STD clinics nationwide.

A second prong of the NCSD program is the development and distribution of publications covering factual issues about the nature of STDs, their prevention, and their treatment. Among these publications is a series of very helpful, one- or two-page charts with detailed information on some specific STD-related issues, such as rapid testing for syphilis, STD program guidelines for policy work and public employees, 2015 CDC STD treatment guidelines, STD contract tracing information, the female condom, and expedited partner therapy.

National Network of STD Clinical Prevention Training Centers

The National Network of STD Clinical Prevention Training Centers (NNPTC) was created in late 2014 as a mechanism for increasing knowledge of health professionals and clinicians about STIs and related issues. The program will run through the end of 2019.

NNPTC has two major components, national and regional. The national component, the National Coordinating Center, aims to ensure uniformity of access and processes among member organizations and individual participants; facilitates resource-sharing among member organizations; oversees and operates the NNPTC website; and aids individual members in dealing with emerging issues in the field. The organization's website also has a mechanism, the Clinical Consultation Service, for answering specific questions from health care professionals about STIs.

The regional component of NNPTC consists of eight training centers distributed around the country for the purpose of providing training in the most recent developments in STI prevention and treatment programs. The centers are located at the St. Louis (Missouri) STD/HIV Prevention Training Center; University of Washington STD Prevention Training Center in Seattle; Alabama–North Carolina STD/HIV Prevention Training Center in Birmingham; STD/HIV Prevention Training

Center at Johns Hopkins University in Baltimore; New York City STD/HIV Prevention Training Center; Sylvie Ratelle STD/HIV Prevention Training Center in Jamaica Plains, Massachusetts; Denver Prevention Training Center; and California Prevention Training Center in Oakland. The programs offered by these centers tend to emphasize clinical and laboratory experience carried out under the guidance of a qualified preceptor. They also offer up-to-date training in fields such as grand rounds, teleconferencing, self-study, on-site courses, and web-based courses.

Albert Ludwig Sigesmund Neisser (1855–1916)

Neisser is best known for his discoveries of the causative agents of two important communicable diseases, gonorrhea and leprosy. In recognition of the first of these achievements, that organism is named in his honor, *Neisseria gonorrhoeae*. (The name was first proposed by Italian bacteriologist Vitorre Trevisan in 1885, although it became widely accepted only about 50 years later.)

Albert Ludwig Sigesmund Neisser (often known as Albert L. Neisser) was born in Scheidnitz, Prussia, near the city of Breslau (now Worclaw, Poland). Neisser attended elementary and high school (gymnasium) in Breslau before matriculating at the University of Breslau in 1872. After a short period of time there, he transferred to the University of Erlagen, from which he received his MD in 1877. Although he had expected to continue his studies in internal medicine, he found the field very crowded and decided to concentrate instead on the field of dermatology. When he completed his medical studies in 1880, he accepted an appointment to the faculty of the University of Leipzig. He spent only two years there before taking a position at the University of Breslau, where he spent the rest of his academic career.

Neisser's work on STDs arose because of the fact that the field of dermatology at the time was home to studies of the subject. Academic departments dealing with the topic were often called the school (or department) of dermatology and venereology. Both of Neisser's historic discoveries were made while he was still a resident at Leipzig. In the case of gonorrhea, he was able to show that a specific organism was responsible for the disease and to isolate and stain the organism. At this point, he suggested the name of *gonococcus* for the organism. In the same year that he made his gonococcus discoveries, Neisser was able to identify the bacillus responsible for leprosy. (That disease is now much better known as Hansen's disease, named for the Norwegian physician Armaur Hansen, who had first isolated the causative agent from tissue taken from leprosy patients.)

Neisser's long and eminent career at Breslau was marred late in his lifetime when he injected four students—without their knowledge or consent—with the spirochete *T. pallidum* in an effort to produce immunity to syphilis. The experiment failed, and all four students eventually developed the disease.

In spite of this unhappy event, Neisser remained a giant in his field, not only pushing the boundaries of STI research, but also working to develop the professional setting in which others in his field could flourish. In 1899, he cofounded the German Dermatological Society and, in 1902, the German Society for Combating Venereal Disease. Late in his life, he worked with Paul Ehrlich, a friend from the Breslau gymnasium, to develop the first reliable cure for syphilis, arsphenamine (salvarsan). Neisser died in Breslau on July 30, 1916, from septicemia, brought on as a result of surgery for kidney disorders from which he had suffered for some time.

Hideyo Noguchi (1876–1928)

In 1913, Noguchi was able to demonstrate that the spirochete bacterium called *T. pallidum* is responsible for syphilis. He made the discovery by identifying the microbe in the brain of patients with paresis, a mental disorder common among individuals in the third stage of syphilis. The bacterium causes widespread damage to brain tissues that manifests as a range of mental disorders.

Noguchi was born Seisaku Noguchi on November 24, 1876, in Inawashiro, Fukushima prefecture, Japan. At the age of 1½ years, he fell into a fireplace, badly burning his left hand. The injury was to have significance on a number of occasions later in life. For example, when the damage to his burned fingers was finally repaired, he was so deeply impressed that he decided to become a physician himself. He apprenticed himself to the doctor who had repaired his hand and eventually passed the medical examination which earned him his MD in 1897. A year later, he changed his name from Seisaku to Hideyo because of a novel he had read about a physician with less than desirable qualities who had the same name as his own birth name.

In 1900, Noguchi took a research position at the University of Pennsylvania, reportedly because prospective employers in Japan were concerned about patient reactions to a doctor with such a badly damaged hand. Noguchi found research a very satisfying career, and later moved from Pennsylvania to a similar position at the Rockefeller Institute in New York City. It was at Rockefeller that Noguchi found the *T. pallidum* bacterium in the brain of a patient with late-term syphilis, providing the evidence that the bacterium was responsible for the disease. For his work in this area, Noguchi was nominated for a Nobel Prize on nine occasions, although he was never given the award.

Beginning in 1918, Noguchi developed a growing interest in yellow fever, and he traveled extensively in South and Central America to test his hypothesis that the disease is caused by a spirochete bacteria like *T. pallidum* rather than by a virus, as most researchers thought (Noguchi was wrong in this hypothesis). While working in Accra, Gold Coast (now Ghana), in 1928, he fell ill with the disease he was studying, and died there on May 21, 1928. He received a number of honors during his lifetime, including the Order of Dannebrog (Denmark), Order of Isabella the Catholic (Spain), Order of the Polar Star

(Sweden), and Order of the Rising Sun, 4th class (Japan); as well as honorary doctorates from the University of Quito, University of Guayaquil, and Yale University. In July 2006, the Japanese government established the Hideyo Noguchi Africa Prize for outstanding research on infectious diseases in Africa.

Thomas J. Parran Jr. (1892–1968)

Parran served as sixth surgeon general of the United States from 1936 to 1948. He was an outspoken advocate of education about STIs (then called venereal diseases) and was very influential in changing public and medical attitudes about the need to talk about, conduct research on, and find solutions to problems related to STIs.

Thomas Parran was born on September 28, 1892, on his parents' tobacco farm near the small town of St. Leonard, Maryland. He was home-schooled by a relative and matriculated at St. John's College in Annapolis, Maryland, with his education being paid for by a scholarship he had earned. He received his bachelor's degree from St. John's in 1911, and his master's four years later. He then continued his studies at Georgetown University, in Washington, D.C., from which he received his MD degree in 1915 also. He completed his internship at the Sibley Memorial Hospital in Washington.

After completing his formal training, Parran was commissioned an assistant surgeon in the PHS, and in 1917 was assigned to the agency's Hygienic Laboratory (later, the NIH). Over the next few years, he was sent to take part in a variety of projects around the country, including research on rural sanitation systems in the South (which involved his role in the construction of new privies for residents there). He also worked on similar projects in other locations such as the health divisions at Fort Oglethorp in Chattanooga, Tennessee; the Muscle Shoals Nitrate Plant near Florence, Alabama; and the Tri-State Sanitary District in Joplin, Missouri, as well as a number of state and local health departments in the South and West.

In late 1923, Parran took part in training classes at PHS headquarters in Washington, where he eventually received the equivalent of a master's degree. Three years later, he was appointed to his first administrative post, as head of the PHS Division of Venereal Diseases. The position stirred his interest in a topic that remained the primary campaign for the rest of his life. He set out to make the public, researchers, and policy makers aware of the challenges posed by gonorrhea and syphilis and worked to gain increased funding for research and education in these areas.

In 1930, New York governor Franklin D. Roosevelt asked the PHS to loan Parran to the state for a period of time to help deal with the crisis created by the Great Depression of the time. Parran made a number of suggestions to deal with the problem, although few were ultimately enacted. It was during this period, however, that a specific event occurred that was to inspire Parran even more strongly to carry on his work in the field of STIs. In November 1934, the Columbia Broadcasting System (CBS) had asked Parran to present a talk about the work of the PHS in the field of infectious diseases. Just moments before the program was to begin, producers of the program reminded Parran that he would not be allowed to use the words *gonorrhea* or *syphilis* on air. In retrospect, the notice should hardly have been surprising to anyone, considering that such terms were considered to be "immoral" and "indecent"; Parran refused to accept the limitation, however, and the broadcast never took place. Biographers have noted that the experience convinced Parran more than ever of removing the veil of secrecy surrounding discussions of STIs.

After Roosevelt became president, he asked Parran to follow him to Washington, where he served on the national Committee on Economic Security, which was later to draft the nation's modern social security system in 1935. When Surgeon General Hugh Cummings's term came to an end a year later, Roosevelt appointed Parran to the position, one in which he served through the first three terms of Roosevelt's administration. He retired on October 1, 1948, to take the position of dean of the new School of Public Health at the University of Pittsburgh. He served in Pittsburgh for 10 years, before retiring and joining the Avalon Foundation, a charitable trust associated with the Mellon Foundation. Parran died in Pittsburgh on February 16, 1968. As one of his biographers has written,

> He, more than any single other person, ushered in what we have come to know as the modern era of STD control and prevention and provided a paradigmatic example of how scientific rigor, excellence, and commitment can be translated into meaningful public policy and action. (Stoner, Bradley P., and Jeanne M. Marrazzo. 2013. "American Sexually Transmitted Diseases Association and the Thomas Parran Award: Past, Present, and Future." *Sexually Transmitted Diseases*, 40(4): 275)

And that would normally have been the conclusion of a productive and admired career in public health service, particularly in the field of STIs. Parran's name resurfaced in 2013, however, when it was revealed that he had been intimately involved with research on the effects of STIs by intentionally inoculating groups of individuals with the causative agents of syphilis and gonorrhea, without their consent, in order to study the effects of the diseases and possible mechanisms for treating the infections. Those studies had been carried out primarily in Guatemala, where restrictions on experiments with humans were, unlike the case in the United States, essentially unregulated. That news prompted the ASTDA to reconsider its actions of many years earlier when it had named its highest award in his honor. On the one hand, some members were willing to forgive Parran in view of his enormous contributions to their field. As one member wrote, "I am confident that if Dr. Parran was around today, he certainly would not approve of or participating in any research work that would even remotely resemble what happened in Guatemala." Other members were not so willing to "forgive and forget." One, for example, wrote that the whole case "reflects at best an overweening belief in one's right to determine that the potential for 'greater good' as the result of a clinical research project justifies trampling individual rights. At worst it reflects racism." In any case, by a vote of 80–20 percent, ASTDA members decided to rename the award as "The ASTDA Distinguished Career Award."

Planned Parenthood

The history of Planned Parenthood is now relatively well known among the general public. On October 16, 1916, a nurse by the name of Margaret Sanger, her sister Ethyl Byrne, and activist Fania Mindell opened a clinic in the Brownsville section of New York City to provide information about birth control, as well as providing birth control devices, such as condoms. More than 100 women took advantage of these services the first day the clinic was open, and about 400 more sought help within the first week. On October 26, however, the New York police raided the clinic and arrested all three women for violating the Comstock Act, formally named the Suppression of Trade in, and Circulation of, Obscene Literature and Articles of Immoral Use. Among the items prohibited from distribution in the act were contraceptives and abortifacients. Upon their release from jail, the three women returned and reopened the clinic on November 16, only to be arrested and jailed a second time. The women persisted in their efforts, and on October 16, 2016, the organization now known as Planned Parenthood celebrated its 100th anniversary.

Today, Planned Parenthood has offices in all 50 states, as well as the District of Columbia. A related organization, the International Planned Parenthood Federation (IPPF), is headquartered in London, with regional offices worldwide in Nairobi, Tunis, Kuala Lumpur, Brussels, New Delhi, and New York. IPPF currently operates in 172 countries with 65,000 discrete service locations, serving more than 90 million individuals annually.

Many people may think of Planned Parenthood as a family planning organization, providing information and services relating to contraception and abortion. Indeed, the intense objection the organization often receives is based on opposition to these practices. In fact, by far the largest portion of its annual budget goes to other types of services, such as body image, cancer issues, men's sexual health, pregnancy, relationships, sexual orientation and gender, women's health, general health care, and STIs. Of its annual budget in 2014–2015, for example, 45 percent went to providing a variety of STI-related services, compared to 31 percent for contraceptive services. Another 13 percent was used for women's health service, 7 percent for cancer screening, and 2 percent for abortion services. The STI services, for example, involved educational information and counseling about early all such diseases, from syphilis, gonorrhea, and chlamydia to pubic lice and scabies. The organization's web page on this topic also includes information about STI testing, including the meaning and practice of safer sex, STI testing, and a tool called "The Check," which helps individuals become aware of the early signs of most STIs. The organization also provides access to online STI testing in three states (Idaho, Minnesota, and Washington), and UTI (urinary tract infection) in these three states plus Alaska, California, and Hawaii. Online testing provides a private conference between individuals and STI experts at remote locations. Presumptive positive indications for an STI can then be followed up with prescription medications sent anonymously to a pharmacy of the patient's preference. The Planned Parenthood website also provides specialized information about STIs for teenagers, parents, and providers.

Project Inform

Project Inform was established in 1984 in San Francisco by Martin Delaney, a consultant to a number of Fortune 500 corporations, and Joe Brewer, a psychotherapist who was treating a number of AIDS patients at the time. The two created the organization in order to make public information about new drugs that might be useful in the battle against HIV/AIDS. At the time, research on AIDS medications was proceeding slowly, and a number of activists in the community, Delaney and Brewer among them, felt it was essential that people with AIDS should have access to the best and most recent information about advances in the field.

The organization continues in these efforts today, along with expanding its programs to include hepatitis C infections. It continues to provide services for men and women living with AIDS and/or hepatitis C, with much of its work centered on the San Francisco Bay area. In 2016, for example, Project Inform provided free HIV medications to some 38,000 individuals in the region who would otherwise not have access to antiviral drugs because of their cost. At the same time, the organization promotes and provides funding for additional research on HIV and hepatitis C with the optimistic goal of creating the first generation free of the two diseases. Part of these efforts involved efforts to encourage drug companies to reduce the cost of HIV/AIDS and hepatitis C medications within the bounds of making a reasonable profit.

Among the tools developed by Project Inform for expanding education about HIV/AIDS and hepatitis C are the electronic newsletter "PiPerspectives News"; a number of publications on pre-exposure prophylaxis; HIV health and wellness booklets; booklets on HIV and hepatitis C coinfections; a screening toolkit about HIV and hepatitis C infections for individuals at risk for the disease and the general public; and a publication explaining coverage available to California residents through state law. Project Inform also provides two help lines about HIV and hepatitis C infections, at 800-822-7422 and 877-435-7443, respectively.

In 2015, the most recent year for which data are available, the organization took in just over $3.287 million, of which more than half came from special events. Another $883,026 came in the form of state and local grants. The organization spent about equal amounts on its regular programs ($1.145 million) and fund-raising ($1.304 million).

Philippe Ricord (1800–1889)

Ricord was a well-known and highly respected French physician and eminent venereologist (a physician who studies venereal diseases). Among his many accomplishments, he is perhaps best known today for his 1838 book, *Traité pratique des maladies vénériennes* (*Practical Work on Venereal Diseases*). He was especially interested in advancing human knowledge of syphilis and outlined his major objectives in the book, namely:

- to prove the existence of a specific cause of syphilitic diseases;
- to distinguish between diseases which resembled each other;
- to establish the differences between primary and generalized syphilitic infection;
- to improve treatment and, if possible, prophylaxis;
- to consider public health and legal aspects of syphilis (J. D. Oriel. 1989. "Eminent Venereologists. 3. Philippe Ricord." *Genitourinary Medicine*, 65: 388–393).

The 19th century saw a vigorous debate among venereologists as to the relationship among syphilis, gonorrhea, and other STIs. One group of specialists, called the *unitarians*, believed that all types of STIs were manifestations of a single disease, syphilis. In the late 1700s, English physician John Hunter had attempted to prove this theory by inoculating a person (some say himself) with the fluid from a syphilitic lesion, after which he developed both syphilis and gonorrhea. In contrast to this view, another group of experts, the *dualists*, believed the syphilis and gonorrhea were distinct diseases. In a series of elegant experiments, Ricord provided conclusive proof that the dualist view of the diseases was more likely correct.

Philippe Ricord was born in Baltimore, Maryland, on December 10, 1800, to parents who had left their native France to escape the worst outrages of the French Revolution. His father died at an early age, and Philippe and his brother, Alexander, were brought up by an older brother. The family struggled to survive, with Philippe having to forego his educational program to take a job as a druggist. In 1820, Philippe and Alexander emigrated to France, where both were offered positions of curators of plant and animal specimens, a career in which Alexander was interested, but not Philippe. His goal was to become a physician, and so he accepted an appointment in 1821 as an extern (an unpaid medical assistant) at the Hospital du Val-de-Grâce in Paris. He soon took a position as an assistant to the well-known French physician, Guillaume Dupuytren. That job also lasted a short time because of personality differences between the two men. He was allowed to continue his medical studies, however, and in 1826, he was granted his MD from the Hopital de la Pitie.

Ricord had difficulty in finding a job after graduation, and eventually had to establish his own practice in a rural area near Orléans. By 1831, he had been offered a job at l'Hopital du Midi, in Paris, an institution that specialized in the treatment of venereal diseases. Ricord had no special training in the field, but rapidly became fascinated by the research challenges it posed. He spent the next 30 years working at Midi, during which time he gained considerable fame as both a researcher and a teacher. One of his biographers, Oriel, has called Ricord "urbane and gregarious" and "one of the most charismatic men of the nineteenth century." In 1892, the Midi hospital where he spent essentially all of his working life was renamed in his honor, Hôpital Ricord. He was also elected president of the Academy of Medicine in 1868, and named honorary chairman of the International Congress of Dermatology and Syphilology in 1889. He continued to work and write until almost his dying day, October 21, 1889, in Paris, where he had also spent most of his life.

Fritz Schaudinn (1871–1906)

Schaudinn was born on September 19, 1871, in Röseningken, East Prussia. He was the only son of an East Prussian family of farmers who showed an interest in the natural sciences at an early age. As is the case with many scientists, he began collecting, displaying, and categorizing plants, insects, and small animals while still quite young. His primary and secondary education took place in the towns of Insterburg and Gumbinnen, now Chernvakhovsk and Gusev, Russia, respectively. He matriculated at the University of Berlin in 1890, planning to concentrate in philosophy. Before long, however, his early interest in the natural sciences caused him to change his mind, and he switched his major to zoology, where he concentrated on the study of protozoa.

After earning his doctorate in 1894, Schaudinn joined a now-famous scientific expedition to Bergen, Norway, where he studied Arctic fauna. At the conclusion of that expedition, he returned to Berlin, where he accepted an appointment as a research assistant at the Zoological Institute of the University of Berlin. In 1898, Schaudinn presented his doctoral thesis to his advisors at Berlin and was granted the degree of privatdozent, an honor somewhat similar to a PhD, which acknowledges a person's expertise in some specific field and allows him or her to teach in that field. In the same year, he took part in a second expedition for the study of Arctic plant life.

In 1901, Schaudinn was appointed director of a German-Austrian research station at Rovigno (now Rovinj, Croatia). The next three years turned out to be, according to one biographer, "the most productive period" in his life. These studies included investigations into the nature, cause, and transmission of malaria, tropical dysentery, trypanosomiasis, and other infective diseases. In 1904, he left Rovigno to assume the post of director of the newly created Institute of Protozoology at the Imperial Ministry of Health in Berlin. His first assignment there was a study of hookworm disease, a condition that had become endemic among German coal miners.

After completing his hookworm studies, Schaudinn turned to a problem involving the causative agent of syphilis. The problem was one that had captured the interest of a number of researchers, but that had thus far escaped resolution. Working with dermatologist Erich Hoffmann at the Charité Hospital in Berlin, Schaudinn eventually discovered a spiral-shaped organism that appeared to be present in syphilitic lesions. They called the new organism *Spirochaeta pallida* ("pale coiled hair"), a name that was later changed to its modern designation of *T. pallidum*. Schaudinn remained very cautious as to asserting that the organism was the actual causative agent of the disease, and still had many critics at the time of his death shortly after the discovery.

In 1906, Schaudinn was appointed the post of director of the newly created Research Institute for Maritime and Tropical Disease in Hamburg. He was at the time, however, already suffering from a condition known as furunculosis that causes painful, pus-filled pustules in the infected area. The disease caused an anal fistula that soon became infected, and he died after returning from an international medical congress in Portugal on June 22, 1906, in Hamburg. Shortly after his death, a fund was created by the German Dermatological Society to honor his discoveries in the field of microbiology. Schaudinn had also been honored with election to the Senckenbergische Naturforschende Gesellschaft (1903), the Imperial Academy of Sciences in St. Petersburg (1905), and the Berlin Society of Internal Medicine (1906).

Sexuality Information and Education Council of the United States

The Sexuality Information and Education Council of the United States (SEICUS) was founded in 1964 by Dr. Mary Calderone, Wallace Fulton, Rev. William Genne, Lester Kirkendall, Dr. Harold Lief, and Clark Vincent for the purpose of providing more complete and more accurate information about human sexuality for adults, children, and teenagers in the United States. Seed money for the new organization was provided by Hugh Hefner, publisher of *Playboy* magazine, who believed in the goals for which SEICUS had been formed. Over the decades, the organization had taken a number of steps to achieve its basic objectives, such as publication of the popular *SEICUS Reports*, a newsletter that provides information about all aspects of human sexuality including current developments in the field; cosponsorship of the advocacy and educational group Gay Men's Health Crisis during the rise of the HIV/AIDS crisis in the mid-1980s as well as publication of the first book for the general public about the disease, *How to Talk to Your Children about AIDS*; an increased interest in advocacy and lobbying of the U.S. Congress and other legislative groups about needed programs in the area of human sexuality in the 1990s; creation of an international arm of the organization at about the same time; and creation of the group's website in 1996.

Current issues in which SEICUS is most interested are comprehensive sex education in the United States; evaluation of abstinence-only-until-marriage sex education programs; adolescent sexuality; teenage pregnancy; STDs; sexual orientation; and sexual and reproductive health. For each of these areas of concern, the organization provides a variety of fact sheets, resources for educators, policy resources, information on research, community action updates, and external links. The SEICUS website is a particularly valuable source of information on topics within these areas, such as fact sheets on the Healthy Youth Act; President Obama's President's Teen Pregnancy Prevention Initiative; status of the recently adopted Personal Responsibility Education Program; public opinion about the status of sex education programs in the United States; status reviews of sex education programs in all 50 states; reviews of state legislation on sex education; and country profiles, policy updates, and other information on sex education in other nations of the world.

Other books, articles, and other resources available from the center include *Guidelines for Comprehensive Sexuality Education: Kindergarten–12th Grade*; a handbook, *Developing Guidelines for Comprehensive Sexuality Education*; a teacher's manual, *Filling the Gaps: Hard-to-Teach Topics in Sexuality Education*; a guide for youth-serving organizations, *On the Right Track?*; a framework for child care centers, *Right from the Start: Guidelines for Sexuality Issues, Birth to Five Years*; a book for young people, *Talk about Sex?*; and two specialized bibliographies, *Sexuality and Disabilities Bibliography* and *Sexuality in Mid- and Later Life Bibliography*.

Stanislaus Josef Mathias von Prowazek (1875–1915)

Von Prowazek is best known today for his contribution (along with Ludwig Halberstädter) to the discovery of the causative agent of chlamydia, an organism now called *C. trachomatis*. In addition to this specific contribution to an understanding of STIs, von Prowazek's work in the field of protistiology (the study of protists) has long been highly regarded. His biographer has called him "one of the most versatile protistologists of his time, both of inconspicuous unicells in the environment and of pathogenic parasites of animal and man."

Prowazek was born on November 12, 1875, in Neuhaus, Böhmen (Bohemia), now Jindřichův Hradec, Bohemia, Czech Republic. His family came from a simple Czech peasant background, whose status was raised when his father was ennobled for his service to the Austro-Hungarian army in 1893. (Ennoblement allows a person to add the honorific "von" to the family name.) At the time, Prowazek himself was a student at the Pizen Gymnasium, where he had changed his name for the traditional family name of Provázek to von Prowazek.

Von Prowazek matriculated at the University of Prague in 1895, where he encountered two teachers who were to become very influential in his life: zoologist Berthold Hatschek, who became von Prowazek's mentor in the field of science, and the physicist and philosopher of science, Ernst Mach, who directed his attention to important issues on the cusp of the interaction between science and society. Because of his attachment to Hatschek, von Prowazek left Prague in 1897 to follow his mentor to his new post at the University of Vienna, from which he received his PhD in protistology in 1899. He then continued to work with Hatschek in Vienna and at the Trieste Zoological Station until 1901.

At that point, von Prowazek was offered the opportunity of working with one of the world's greatest researchers in biology at the time, Paul Ehrlich, at Ehrlich's Institute for Experimental Therapy in Frankfurt. Two years later, he left the institute to join a research team at the University of Berlin at Rovigno, where he joined a colleague from the Trieste station, Fritz Schaudinn. The move brought together two researchers who were each to make critical breakthroughs in the history of STIs: Schaudinn was to discover the causative agent of syphilis, *T. pallidum*, in 1905, and von Prowazek, who was to make a similar discovery for chlamydia in 1907.

Schaudinn's and von Prowazek's careers remained intertwined after the former was named director of the zoological section at the Institut für Schiffs- und Tropenkrankheiten (Institute for Maritime and Tropical Medicine) in Hamburg in 1905. After only a year at the helm, Schaudinn died, and von Prowazek was appointed his successor. For essentially the rest of his life, von Prowazek traveled throughout the world pursuing his research on a variety of infectious diseases: to Java with Neisser to study gonorrhea; to Batavia for the study of trachoma; to Brazil for the study of vaccinia and variola; to the western Pacific to study trachoma and a variety of other diseases; and to Serbia and Constantinople to study typhus. His last project concerned an epidemic that had broken out among Russian prisoners housed in the German city of Cottbus during World War I. Both he and a fellow researcher, H. T. Ricketts, eventually died of the disease, von Prowazek in Cottbus on February 17, 1915. A third colleague, Henrique

Da Rocha-Lima, survived the disease, discovered the causative agent, and named that agent in honor of his two dead friends, *Rickettsia prowazekii*.

August Paul von Wassermann (1866–1925)

Von Wassermann's fame in the history of venereology rests on his discovery in 1906 of a method for testing to see if a person had been infected with the *T. pallidum* bacterium that causes syphilis. That development occurred only a year after the discovery itself that the microorganism was the causative agent in the disease. The test, subsequently known as the Wassermann test, was of inestimable value because the early stages of syphilis are sometimes asymptomatic, and it may be difficult for an individual to know that he or she has been infected. But one of the important features of treatment for syphilis is early diagnosis so that a treatment regimen can be started as soon as possible. The technology used by Wassermann in his research is known as complement fixation, a method by which antitoxins or antigens in a person's body can be detected by the reaction between an added reagent and a sample of the patient's blood.

August Paul von Wassermann was born in Bamberg, Germany, on February 21, 1866, to Angelo and Dora (Bauer) Wassermann. His father was a banker to the court of Bavaria and for his services was awarded in 1909 with the honorary title of "von" to be added to the family name. August had his primary and secondary education in Bamberg, and then continued his studies at the universities of Erlangen, Vienna, Munich, and Strassburg, from which he received his medical degree in 1888. In 1891, he took a position as an unpaid assistant at the newly created Institute for Infectious Diseases in Berlin, created by the eminent microbiologist Roberg Koch. At the institute, Wassermann was assigned work on problems related to cholera and was made inspecting physician at the institute's antitoxin control station for diphtheria. In 1901, he was named privat-dozent at the Friedrich Wilhelm University in Berlin, a title that provided a comfortable salary and the right to teach classes in his area of expertise. He was later promoted to the post of professor extraordinarius (extraordinary professor) that allowed him time to focus on his research. In 1906, he was also named director of the division of experimental therapy and serum research at the Institute for Infectious Diseases. A year later, he was named Geheimer Medizinalrat ("secret medical counselor," a high court position). In 1913, Wassermann left the institute to become director of the Institute for Experimental Therapy at the Kaiser Wilhelm Society for the Advancement of Science in Berlin.

Wassermann's academic career, like that of most of his colleagues, was interrupted by the onset of World War I. He left his position at the Kaiser Wilhelm Society, was appointed a brigadier general in the German army, and was placed in charge of efforts to control infectious disease on the Eastern Front. After the war, he returned to the expanded and renamed Institute for Experimental Therapy and Biochemistry in Berlin as director of the institute. He served for only a brief period of time, however, before he began to suffer from Bright's disease (glomerulonephritis), a condition from which he died in Berlin on March 16, 1925.

Wassermann's work was recognized worldwide, and he received a number of honors and awards from governments and academies in many countries, such as Belgium, Japan, Romania, Spain, Turkey, and his native Prussia. In 1921, he was named the first winner of the Aronson Foundation Prize, awarded biennially for achievements in microbiology and immunology.

Harald zur Hausen (1936–)

Harald zur Hausen is a German virologist who was awarded the 2008 Nobel Prize in physiology or medicine for his discovery of the role of the HPV in cancer of the cervix. His work made possible the eventual development of a vaccine that protects women against HPV and, thus, significantly decreases their risk for both cervical cancer and genital warts.

Harald zur Hausen was born in Gelsenkirchen, Germany, on March 11, 1936. He attended high school in Vechta and then studied medicine at the universities of Bonn, Hamburg, and Düsseldorf, from which he received his MD in 1960. After serving for two years as a medical assistant at Düsseldorf, zur Hausen took a position as a laboratory researcher at the Institute for Microbiology at Düsseldorf. In 1966, he emigrated to the United States to work at the Virus Laboratories of the University of Pennsylvania's Children's Hospital with the famous expatriate German virologists, Werner and Gertrude Henle. In 1969, zur Hausen returned to Germany, where he served successively as professor of virology at the University of Würzburg (1969–1972), the University of Erlangen-Nuremberg (1972–1977), and the University of Freiburg (1977–1983). In 1983, he was appointed director of the German Cancer Research Center (GCRC; Deutsches Krebsforschungszentrum) in Heidelberg and professor of medicine at the University of Heidelberg. In 2003, he retired and was named professor emeritus at the GCRC. Although officially retired, zur Hausen continues (as of 2017) to work at GCRC, heading a research team studying viruses that may be responsible for colorectal cancer.

Zur Hausen became interested in the role of viruses in the development of cancer early in his career. At the time, scientists had found that viruses are responsible for cancer in some animals, but their role in any form of cancer in humans was still unclear. In 1983, zur Hausen discovered the presence of one form of HPV, called HPV 16, in cervical cancer tumors. A year later, he discovered a second type of HPV, HPV 18, in similar cervical tumors. He became convinced that HPV was the causative agent in at least some types of cervical cancers. Zur Hausen's discovery was greeted with serious doubt by most cancer researchers since the predominant theory at the time was that a different type of virus, the one responsible for herpes simplex, was the causative agent in cervical cancer. Evidence for zur Hausen's hypothesis accumulated over the years, however, and there is now no doubt as to the role of HPV in causing both cervical cancer and genital warts. In addition to his Nobel Prize, zur Hausen has received a number of other important awards, including the Robert Koch Prize, Charles S. Mott Prize, Paul-Ehrlich-und-Ludwig-Darmstaedter-Preis, Virchow Medal, San Marino Prize for Medicine, Great Cross of Merit of the Federal Republic of Germany, William B. Coley Award, and Gairdner Foundation International Award.

BEFORE YOU MAKE YOUR MOVE

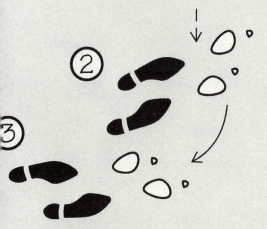

...YOU BETTER KNOW WHAT STEPS TO TAKE.

SOMETIMES THE BEST STEP IS TO
STEP AWAY.

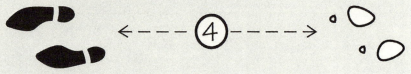

It's the best protection against sexually transmitted disea.

Introduction

This chapter provides two types of research resources for the reader. The first is a set of data tables that contain statistics on the incidence and prevalence of sexually transmitted infections (STIs) in the United States. The second is a sampling of certain important documents dealing with STI issues in the United States. These documents include laws, court cases, and reports that have been issued on the topic.

Data

Table 5.1 Incidence of Certain STIs in the United States, 1941–2015

| | Syphilis | | | | Chlamydia | | Gonorrhea | |
| | All Stages | | Primary and Secondary | | | | | |
Year	Number	Rate[1]	Number	Rate[1]	Number	Rate[1]	Number	Rate[1]
1941	485,560	368.2	68,231	51.7	NR	—	193,468	146.7
1942	479,601	363.4	75,312	57.0	NR	—	212,403	160.9
1943	575,593	447.0	82,204	63.8	NR	—	275,070	213.6
1944	467,755	367.9	78,443	61.6	NR	—	300,676	236.5
1945	359,114	282.3	77,007	60.5	NR	—	287,181	225.8
1946	363,647	271.7	94,957	70.9	NR	—	368,020	275.0

(continued)

A U.S. Department of Defense poster issued during 1988-2000, suggesting abstinence as the best way to prevent sexually transmitted diseases. (Department of Defense)

Table 5.1   (Continued)

Year	Syphilis				Chlamydia		Gonorrhea	
	All Stages		Primary and Secondary					
	Number	Rate[1]	Number	Rate[1]	Number	Rate[1]	Number	Rate[1]
1947	355,592	252.3	93,545	66.4	NR	—	380,666	270.0
1948	314,313	218.2	68,174	47.3	NR	—	345,501	239.8
1949	256,463	175.3	41,942	28.7	NR	—	317,950	217.3
1950	217,558	146.0	23,939	16.7	NR	—	286,746	192.5
1951	174,924	116.1	14,485	9.6	NR	—	254,470	168.9
1952	167,762	110.2	10,449	6.9	NR	—	244,957	160.8
1953	148,573	95.9	8,637	5.6	NR	—	238,340	153.9
1954	130,697	82.9	7,147	4.5	NR	—	242,050	153.5
1955	122,392	76.2	6,454	4.0	NR	—	236,197	147.0
1956	130,201	78.7	6,392	3.9	NR	—	224,346	135.7
1957	123,758	73.5	6,576	3.9	NR	—	214,496	127.4
1958	113,884	66.4	7,176	4.2	NR	—	232,386	135.6
1959	120,824	69.2	9,799	5.6	NR	—	240,254	137.6
1960	122,538	68.8	16,145	9.1	NR	—	258,933	145.4
1961	124,658	68.8	19,851	11.0	NR	—	264,158	145.8
1962	126,245	68.7	21,067	11.5	NR	—	263,714	143.6
1963	124,137	66.5	22,251	11.9	NR	—	278,289	149.0
1964	114,325	60.4	22,969	12.1	NR	—	300,666	158.9
1965	112,842	58.9	23,338	12.2	NR	—	324,925	169.5
1966	105,159	54.2	21,414	11.0	NR	—	351,738	181.2
1967	102,581	52.2	21,053	10.7	NR	—	404,836	205.9
1968	96,271	48.4	19,019	9.6	NR	—	464,543	233.4
1969	92,162	45.7	19,130	9.5	NR	—	534,872	265.4
1970	91,382	44.8	21,982	10.8	NR	—	600,072	294.2
1971	95,997	46.4	23,783	11.5	NR	—	670,268	324.1
1972	91,149	43.6	24,429	11.7	NR	—	767,215	366.6
1973	87,469	41.4	24,825	11.7	NR	—	842,621	398.7
1974	83,771	39.3	25,385	11.9	NR	—	906,121	424.7
1975	80,356	37.3	25,561	11.9	NR	—	999,937	464.1
1976	71,761	33.0	23,731	10.9	NR	—	1,001,994	460.6

| Year | Syphilis | | | | Chlamydia | | Gonorrhea | |
| | All Stages | | Primary and Secondary | | | | | |
	Number	Rate[1]	Number	Rate[1]	Number	Rate[1]	Number	Rate[1]
1977	64,621	29.4	20,399	9.3	NR	—	1,002,219	456.0
1978	64,875	29.2	21,656	9.8	NR	—	1,013,436	456.3
1979	67,049	29.9	24,874	11.1	NR	—	1,004,058	447.1
1980	68,832	30.3	27,204	12.0	NR	—	1,004,029	442.1
1981	72,799	31.7	31,266	13.6	NR	—	990,864	431.8
1982	75,579	32.6	33,613	14.5	NR	—	960,633	414.7
1983	74,637	31.9	32,698	14.0	NR	—	900,435	385.1
1984	69,872	29.6	28,607	12.1	7,594	6.5	878,556	372.5
1985	67,563	28.4	27,131	11.4	25,848	17.4	911,419	383.0
1986	67,779	28.2	27,667	11.5	58,001	35.2	892,229	371.5
1987	87,286	36.0	35,585	14.7	91,913	50.8	787,532	325.0
1988	104,546	42.8	40,474	16.6	157,854	87.1	738,160	301.9
1989	115,089	46.6	45,826	18.6	200,904	102.5	733,294	297.1
1990	135,590	54.3	50,578	20.3	323,663	160.2	690,042	276.4
1991	128,719	50.9	42,950	17.0	381,228	179.7	621,918	245.8
1992	114,730	44.7	34,009	13.3	409,694	182.3	502,858	196.0
1993	102,612	39.5	26,527	10.2	405,332	178.0	444,649	171.1
1994	82,713	31.4	20,641	7.8	451,785	192.5	419,602	163.9
1995	69,359	26.0	16,543	6.2	478,577	187.8	392,651	147.5
1996	53,240	19.8	11,405	4.2	492,631	190.6	328,169	121.8
1997	46,716	17.1	8,556	3.1	537,904	205.5	327,665	120.2
1998	38,289	13.9	7,007	2.5	614,250	231.8	356,492	129.2
1999	35,386	12.7	6,617	2.4	662,647	247.2	360,813	129.3
2000	31,618	11.2	5,979	2.1	709,452	251.4	363,136	128.7
2001	32,286	11.3	6,103	2.1	783,242	274.5	361,705	126.8
2002	32,919	11.4	6,862	2.4	834,555	289.4	351,852	122.0
2003	34,289	11.8	7,177	2.5	877,478	301.7	335,104	115.2
2004	33,423	11.4	7,980	2.7	929,462	316.5	330,132	112.4
2005	33,288	11.2	8,724	2.9	976,445	329.4	339,593	114.6
2006	36,958	12.3	9,756	3.3	1,030,911	344.3	358,366	119.7
2007	40,925	13.6	11,466	3.8	1,108,374	367.5	355,991	118.0

(continued)

Table 5.1   (Continued)

Year	Syphilis All Stages Number	Rate[1]	Primary and Secondary Number	Rate[1]	Chlamydia Number	Rate[1]	Gonorrhea Number	Rate[1]
2008	46,292	15.2	13,500	4.4	1,210,523	398.1	336,742	110.7
2009	44,832	14.6	13,997	4.6	1,244,180	405.3	301,174	98.1
2010	45,844	14.8	13,774	4.5	1,307,893	423.6	309,341	100.2
2011	46,040	14.8	13,970	4.5	1,412,791	453.4	321,849	103.3
2012	49,915	15.9	15,667	5.0	1,422,976	453.3	334,826	106.7
2013	56,484	17.9	17,375	5.5	1,401,906	443.5	333,004	105.3
2014	63,453	19.9	19,999	6.3	1,441,789	452.2	350,062	109.8
2015	74,702	23.4	23,872	7.5	1,526,658	478.8	395,216	123.9

Source: "Sexually Transmitted Diseases—Reported Cases and Rates of Reported Cases per 100,000 Population, United States, 1941–2015." 2016. Sexually Transmitted Disease Surveillance 2015, Table 1, pages 85–86. https://www.cdc.gov/std/stats15/std-surveillance-2015-print.pdf. Accessed on February 2, 2017.

[1]Per 100,000 population.

NR = not a reportable disease.

Table 5.2   Cases of Chlamydia in the United States, by Age and Sex, 2015

Age Group	Total Number	Rate[1]	Male Number	Rate[1]	Female Number	Rate[1]	Unknown Sex Number
0–4	518	2.6	196	1.9	322	3.3	0
5–9	148	0.7	18	0.2	130	1.3	0
10–14	10,642	51.5	1,216	11.5	9,394	92.8	32
15–19	391,396	1,857.8	82,775	767.6	307,937	2,994.4	684
20–24	589,963	2,574.9	172,313	1,467.8	416,772	3,730.3	878
25–29	280,429	1,275.4	104,679	937.9	175,291	1,619.1	459
30–34	123,866	575.4	52,019	481.3	71,653	668.4	194
35–39	59,905	300.7	27,180	273.4	32,621	326.8	104
40–44	30,379	147.5	15,210	148.8	15,118	145.8	51
45–54	28,833	66.3	17,011	79.4	11,764	53.4	58
55–64	7,756	19.4	4,901	25.4	2,840	13.7	15

Age Group	Total		Male		Female		Unknown Sex
	Number	Rate[1]	Number	Rate[1]	Number	Rate[1]	Number
65+	1,596	3.5	1,043	5.1	546	2.1	7
Unknown	1,227	—	420	—	755	—	52
TOTAL	1,526,658	478.8	478,981	305.2	1,045,143	645.5	2,534

Source: "Chlamydia—Reported Cases and Rates of Reported Cases by Age Group and Sex, United States, 2011–2015." Sexually Transmitted Disease Surveillance 2015, Table 10, page 95. https://www.cdc.gov/std/stats15/std-surveillance-2015-print.pdf. Accessed on February 2, 2017.

[1]Per 100,000.

Table 5.3   Cases of Gonorrhea in the United States, by Age and Sex, 2015

Age Group	Total		Male		Female		Unknown Sex
	Number	Rate[1]	Number	Rate[1]	Number	Rate[1]	
0–4	148	0.7	47	0.5	98	1.0	3
5–9	78	0.4	11	0.1	66	0.7	1
10–14	2,312	11.2	385	3.6	1,923	19.0	4
15–19	72,001	341.8	26,401	244.8	45,477	442.2	123
20–24	124,592	543.8	63,289	539.1	61,105	546.9	198
25–29	82,867	376.9	50,089	448.8	32,662	301.7	116
30–34	45,681	212.2	29,751	275.2	15,867	148.0	63
35–39	26,137	131.2	18,198	183.1	7,897	79.1	42
40–44	15,042	73.0	11,116	108.8	3,898	37.6	28
45–54	18,779	43.2	15,379	71.8	3,375	15.3	25
55–64	6,035	15.1	5,175	26.8	849	4.1	11
65+	1,191	2.6	1,032	5.1	158	0.6	1
Unknown Age	353	—	197	—	139	—	17
TOTAL	395,216	123.9	221,070	140.9	173,514	107.2	632

Source: "Gonorrhea—Reported Cases and Rates of Reported Cases by Age Group and Sex, United States, 2011–2015." Sexually Transmitted Disease Surveillance 2015, Table 21, page 107. https://www.cdc.gov/std/stats15/std-surveillance-2015-print.pdf. Accessed on February 2, 2017.

[1] Per 100,000.

Table 5.4   Cases of Primary and Secondary Syphilis in the United States, by Age and Sex, 2015

Age Group	Total Number	Rate[1]	Male Number	Rate[1]	Female Number	Rate[1]	Unknown Sex
0–4	2	0.0	0	0.0	1	0.0	1
5–9	1	0.0	0	0.0	1	0.0	0
10–14	9	0.0	1	0.0	8	0.1	0
15–19	1,148	5.4	865	8.0	283	2.8	0
20–24	4,766	20.8	4,186	35.7	573	5.1	7
25–29	5,168	23.5	4,671	41.8	491	4.5	6
30–34	3,549	16.5	3,234	29.9	311	2.9	4
35–39	2,482	12.5	2,249	22.6	229	2.3	4
40–44	1,897	9.2	1,744	17.1	152	1.5	1
45–54	3,488	8.0	3,294	15.4	190	0.9	4
55–64	1,153	2.9	1,099	5.7	54	0.3	0
65+	207	0.4	202	1.0	5	0.0	0
Unknown Age	2	—	2	—	0	—	0
TOTAL	23,872	7.5	21,547	13.7	2,298	1.4	27

Source: "Primary and Secondary Syphilis—Reported Cases and Rates of Reported Cases by Age Group and Sex, United States, 2011–2015." Sexually Transmitted Disease Surveillance 2015, Table 34, page 121. https://www.cdc.gov/std/stats15/std-surveillance-2015-print.pdf. Accessed on February 2, 2017.

[1]Per 100,000.

Table 5.5   States with Highest and Lowest Rates of Certain STIs, 2015

Rank	State	Cases	Rate (per 100,000)
Chlamydia			
1	Alaska	5,660	768.3
2	Louisiana	32,325	695.2
3	North Carolina	64,376	647.4
4	New Mexico	12,632	605.7
5	Mississippi	17,371	580.2
6	Georgia	57,639	570.8

Rank	State	Cases	Rate (per 100,000)
7	South Carolina	27,538	569.9
8	Arkansas	16,166	545.0
9	Alabama	26,359	543.6
10	Oklahoma	21,025	542.2
11	Illinois	69,610	540.4
12	New York	103,615	524.7
U.S. total		1,526,658	478.8
48	Utah	8,633	293.3
49	West Virginia	4,958	268.0
50	New Hampshire	3,095	233.3
Gonorrhea			
1	Louisiana	10,282	221.1
2	North Carolina	19,809	199.2
3	Mississippi	5,775	192.9
4	South Carolina	8,206	169.8
5	Oklahoma	6,542	168.7
6	Arkansas	4,780	161.1
7	Georgia	15,982	158.3
8	Alaska	1,113	151.1
9	Alabama	7,196	148.4
10	Missouri	8,942	147.5
11	Texas	39,717	147.3
12	Ohio	16,564	142.9
U.S. total		395,216	123.9
48	Idaho	472	28.9
49	Vermont	155	24.7
50	New Hampshire	245	18.5
Primary and Secondary Syphilis			
1	Louisiana	696	15.0
2	Georgia	1,413	14.0
3	California	4,908	12.6

(continued)

Table 5.5 (Continued)

Rank	State	Cases	Rate (per 100,000)
4	North Carolina	1,196	12.0
5	Nevada	335	11.8
6	Florida	2,083	10.5
7	New York	2,006	10.2
8	Arizona	589	8.7
9	Oregon	345	8.7
10	Maryland	509	8.5
11	Illinois	1,085	8.4
U.S. total		23,872	7.5
12	Mississippi	219	7.3
48	Montana	13	1.3
49	Alaska	8	1.1
50	Wyoming	5	0.9

Source: "Chlamydia/Gonorrhea/Primary and Secondary Syphilis—Reported Cases and Rates of Reported Cases by State, Ranked by Rates, United States, 2015." Sexually Transmitted Disease Surveillance 2015, Tables 2, 13, 26, pages 87, 99, 113. https://www.cdc.gov/std/stats15/std-surveillance-2015-print.pdf. Accessed on February 2, 2017.

Table 5.6　HIV Infection Statistics, United States, 2015

Trait	Number	Rate (per 100,000)[1]
Age		
<13	174	0.3
13–14	35	0.4
15–19	1,828	8.7
20–24	7,868	34.3
25–29	7,870	35.8
30–34	6,026	28.0
35–39	4,662	23.4
40–44	4,196	20.4
45–49	4,021	19.3
50–54	3,242	14.4
55–59	2,166	10.1

Trait	Number	Rate (per 100,000)[1]
60–64	1,069	5.8
>64	914	2.0
Race/ethnicity		
American Indian/Alaska Native	222	9.5
Asian	1,046	6.2
Black/African American	19,540	49.4
Hispanic/Latino	10,201	18.4
Native Hawaiian/Other Pacific Islander	58	10.6
White	12,025	6.1
Multiple races	982	15.4
Method of transmission		
Male		
Male-to-male sexual contact	29,418	−2
Injection drug use	1,590	−2
Both male-to-male sexual contact and injection drug use	1,217	−2
Heterosexual contact	3,285	−2
Other	60	−2
Subtotal	35,571	27.4
Female		
Injection drug use	1,045	−2
Heterosexual contact	7,242	−2
Other	41	−2
Subtotal	8,328	6.1
Child (<13 years of age at diagnosis)		
Perinatal	127	−2
Other	48	−2
Subtotal	174	0.3
Total	44,073	13.8

Source: "Diagnoses of HIV Infection in the United States and Dependent Areas, 2014." HIV Surveillance Report. Volume 26, Table 1a, pages 18–19. https://www.cdc.gov/hiv/pdf/library/reports/surveillance/cdc-hiv-surveillance-report-2014-vol--26.pdf. Accessed on February 2, 2017.

[1]Estimates based on statistical adjustment that account for reporting delays and missing transmission category, but not for incomplete reporting.

[2]Not calculated.

Table 5.7 Prevalence of Any Genital HPV among Adults Aged 18–59

	Any Genital HPV			High Risk Genital HPV		
Group	All	Men	Women	All	Men	Women
Total population	42.5	45.2	39.9	22.7	25.1	20.4
Non-Hispanic Asian	23.8	24.4	23.2	11.9	12.2	11.6
Non-Hispanic white	40.0	43.7	36.5	21.6	24.7	18.7
Non-Hispanic black	64.1	65.0	63.2	33.7	40.3	28.2
All Hispanic	41.4	44.4	38.5	21.7	21.8	21.6

Source: McQuillan, Geraldine, et al. 2017. "Prevalence of HPV in Adults Aged 18–69: United States, 2011–2014." Centers for Disease Control and Prevention, Figures 3 and 4. https://www.cdc.gov/nchs/data/databriefs/db280_table.pdf#1. Accessed on April 9, 2017.

Documents

BN v. KK (1988)

One of the most fundamental legal questions associated with STIs has to do with the responsibility that one person may have for a second person's physical, mental, and emotional health as the result of sexual intercourse between the two. One of the earliest cases of this type was adjudicated in 1988. It involved a nurse (BN) who became involved in a relationship with a doctor with whom she worked (KK). KK had, at the time of the relationship, a case of genital herpes, which he failed to mention to BN. When BN also contracted herpes, she sued KK for withholding this information from her during the relationship. The U.S. District Court for the District of Maryland asked the Court of Appeals of Maryland for advice on the legal standing of the defendant. The Court of Appeals then laid out the challenge it confronted. (Triple asterisks [***] indicate omitted references.)

Does Maryland Recognize A Cause of Action for Either Fraud, Intentional Infliction Of Emotional Distress, Or Negligence Resulting From the Sexual Transmission Of A Dangerous, Contagious, and Incurable Disease, Such As Genital Herpes?

. . .

On the basis of these general allegations, as well as some others contained in particular counts, to some of which we shall later refer, Ms. N. charged Dr. K. with fraud (count one); intentional infliction of emotional distress (count two); negligence (count three); and assault and battery (count four).

After reviewing the evidence, the court then states its decision on each of the four counts:

[Negligence] . . . Ms. N. has alleged that Dr. K., knowing he had active genital herpes, a highly contagious, sexually transmitted disease, had sexual intercourse with her. *** If she can prove these allegations, it would be reasonably foreseeable by Dr. K. (or a fact-finder could so conclude) that Ms. N. would be harmed by his conduct. She was a clearly identified potential victim. *** As a consequence, Dr. K. had a duty either to refrain from sexual contact with Ms. N. or to warn her of his condition. If, as she charges, he negligently failed to do either, he breached his duty.

. . . *[Infliction of Emotional Distress]* . . . Ms. N. avers, in her emotional distress count, that Dr. K., aware of the fact that he had active genital herpes, a contagious and incurable disease that is spread by sexual contact, engaged in sexual intercourse with her, thereby transmitting the disease to her. These allegations suffice, if established, to support the first element of the tort.

Even if Dr. K. did not actually intend to inflict severe emotional distress, it is enough if "he [knew] that such distress [was] certain, or substantially certain, to result from his conduct; or where [he acted] recklessly in deliberate disregard of a high degree of probability that the emotional distress [would] follow."*** This is so because according to the facts we must take as established for the purposes of this case, Dr. K. knew the nature of the disease, including its painful nature and its incurability, and also that his disease was active at the time he had sex with Ms. N., and that the disease, in its active state, is transmitted through sexual intercourse.*** That the transmission of genital herpes is substantially certain to produce severe emotional distress appears from the characteristics of the illness; these characteristics also support the extreme and outrageous nature of Dr. K.'s conduct, if they are adequately proven.

. . .

On the record before us and in a case of this type, we obviously cannot pass on the sufficiency of the evidence as to the severity of Ms. N.'s emotional distress. We can only hold, as we do, that proof of acts such as those we have outlined establish the first three elements of the tort of intentional infliction of emotional distress under Maryland law. If sufficiently severe emotional distress has been produced by that conduct, in light of all the evidence, Ms. N. is entitled to recover.

. . . *[Fraud]* Whether Ms. N. reasonably relied upon the implicit representation of good health that resulted from Dr. K.'s nondisclosure is a question of fact depending to some degree on the nature of their relationship; she has alleged reasonable reliance. The implicit misrepresentation was obviously a material one; Ms. N. asserts that she never would have engaged in sex with Dr. K. had she known the truth; she also avers that she suffered damage directly from the misrepresentation. Consequently, she has also stated a cause of action for fraud that is recognized in Maryland.

Source: *BN v. KK*, 538 A.2d 1175 (Md. 1988).

GL v. ML (1988)

One of the major changes in case law with regard to liability for the transmission of an STI has to do with such events within a legal marriage. For most of U.S. history, the courts have ruled that husbands and wives could not sue each other for actions that might otherwise be illegal outside a legal marriage. In many cases, that doctrine was based on the principle that wives are the property of their husbands and have no independent legal rights. In other cases, courts have ruled that legal proceedings within a marriage might destroy the "sanctity" of such a relationship. (For an extended discussion of this point, see James B. Damiano. 2012. "Sexually Transmitted Diseases: A Courtroom Epidemic." Law School Student Scholarship. http://scholarship.shu.edu/cgi/viewcontent.cgi?article=1021&conte xt=student_scholarship. Accessed on February 6, 2017. And note in particular the title of the article.) This trend began to change after 1960, and, although the courts are not yet unanimous in their stand on the issue, the rights of women to sue their husbands is now a well-established legal principle in most states.

The case cited here is one of a series of similar suits processed through the courts of New Jersey in the 1970s and 1980s that have established a precedent for suits by individuals who contracted an STI from their spouse within a marriage. One of the most important of those cases has been GL v. ML, discussed here. The court's decision begins with the court's review of the facts in the case. (Triple asterisks [***] indicate the omission of certain citations.)

The plaintiff in this matter filed for divorce on November 2, 1984. Included in her complaint were four separate counts for personal injury alleging that her husband, the defendant, transmitted genital herpes to her during their marriage. . . .

In the present action, the plaintiff alleges that the defendant continued to have sexual relations with her even after discovering that he had herpes, the result of an extramarital relationship. It is argued by the defendant that sexual intercourse between spouses is by its very nature an act which falls within the scope of a marital or nuptial privilege and therefore his conduct should be shielded from liability. . . .

[The court then explains its verdict.]

This Court does not agree. It is unconscionable that a person could escape liability for infecting a spouse with genital herpes or other sexually transmitted disease by merely claiming that the transmission occurred during privileged sexual relations of marriage. As early as Crowell v. Crowell, 180 N.C. 516, 105 S.E. 206 (Sup.Ct. 1920), reh. den. 181 N.C. 66, 106 S.E. 149 (Sup.Ct. 1921), courts began to recognize a cause of action in tort for the transmission of venereal disease to one's spouse.

Defendant misconstrues the meaning of marital privilege and furthermore destroyed any that may have existed by his own intentional involvement in an extramarital relationship. Defendant cannot simultaneously breach his marital relationship by engaging in extramarital intercourse, and claim nuptial immunity for consequences flowing from his own wilful and *** intentional conduct.

. . .

There remains a duty of care to one's spouse and the threat of physical harm cannot be excused. . . . Although a criminal charge is not being addressed, the defendant can not be allowed to hide behind the veil of marital privilege.

Decisions within our own state and those in other parts of the nation provide no justification to bar this suit on the basis of interspousal immunity. . . .

This Court holds that the marital privilege of sexual relations does not include immunity to personal injury suits between spouses based upon the transmittal of a sexual disease.

Source: *GL v. ML*, 550 A.2d 525 (N.J. Super. Ct. App. Div. 1988).

Doe v. Roe (1990)

One of the most contentious issues in case law with regard to STIs has to do with the legal responsibility of either or both of two individuals involved in a sexual relationship in which one has an STI. That is, if A and B are having sexual intercourse with each other (once or on a number of occasions), is A or B required to inform his or her partner that he or she may have syphilis, gonorrhea, chlamydia, herpes, or some other STI? A variety of courts have ruled on this question, generally with a "yes" as their answer (although some exceptions have occurred). Typical of this response is a decision of the California Court of Appeal in 1990, as outlined below. (Triple asterisks [***] indicate the omission of citations.)

[The court first reviews the circumstances of the case:]

Defendant and plaintiff became acquainted in early 1985 while working together at a supermarket. Defendant asked her out several times and they engaged in frank and open discussions about sexual intercourse and other personal matters. Defendant told her that he had been involved in a long-time relationship with his live-in girlfriend and plaintiff told him she was involved with a boyfriend who was a merchant marine and away at sea. Soon after he asked her out, the subject of venereal disease came up. Plaintiff told defendant that she and her boyfriend were "clean," and that she would not want to put herself in a position where she could possibly contract a sexual disease. Defendant replied, "I don't blame you, I wouldn't want one either," but did not tell her he had previously contracted herpes.

In fact, defendant had suffered three prior outbreaks of herpes.

. . .

[The court then explains a major portion of its decision:]

The evidence shows defendant knew he had herpes and that it could be transmitted by sexual contact. Although he had several outbreaks of the virus prior to 1985, defendant did absolutely nothing to find out about its contagiousness or what steps could be taken to prevent his giving it to a prospective partner. Defendant also testified that his lesions would appear*** at times without warning. Knowing that he had this infectious condition and that plaintiff was concerned about contracting venereal disease, defendant entered into a sexual liaison with plaintiff and continued to have intercourse with her on a regular basis for four months without revealing to her this material fact, electing to gamble with her health rather than inform her of his condition or educate himself about the disease. Under these facts, the record supports the court's implied finding that the risk of harm was foreseeable and that defendant unreasonably failed to exercise due care to guard against this risk.***

"A reasonable person should know that if he/she has a contagious, sexually transmissible disease like genital herpes, the disease is likely to be communicated through sexual contact. Thus people suffering from genital herpes generally have a duty either to avoid sexual contact with uninfected persons or, at least to warn potential sex partners that they have herpes before sexual contact occurs." ***

(1d) Our conclusion is not altered by the fact that defendant did not have an active outbreak of the disease during the relationship. There is no evidence in the record to support defendant's repeated assertion that he "relied on his doctors," in failing to disclose the condition or take precautionary measures during sex. No one, much less a physician, told plaintiff that he could not transmit herpes as long he did not have lesions; defendant simply made up his mind that such was the case.

Source: *Doe v. Roe*, 218 Cal. App. 3d 1538 (Cal. Ct. App. 1990).

United States v. Staff Sergeant Adolphus A. Young (2016)

One of the most common prosecutions involving STIs involves cases in which an individual who is HIV positive has sexual intercourse with someone who is HIV negative and unaware of his or her partner's HIV status. The Center for HIV Law and Policy maintains an ongoing list of such cases and recently posted a list of 279 such cases that had reached the courts between 2008 and 2016 (http://www.hivlawandpolicy.org/resources/prosecutions-and-arrests-hiv-exposure-united-states-2008%E2%80%932016-list-center-hiv-law-policy). One such case taken from that list has the added component of involving a member of the armed services who admitted to having sexual relationships with a number of partners, at least some of whom were not aware of his HIV status. The circumstances of that case and the military court's decision with regard to it are as follows.

In accordance with his pleas, Appellant was convicted of four specifications of willful dereliction of duty for failing to inform sexual partners of his human immunodeficiency virus (HIV) positive status and engaging in unprotected sexual activity, two specifications of assault consummated by a battery for having oral and anal intercourse without disclosing his HIV-positive status, and one specification of obstruction of justice, in violation of Articles 92, 128, and 134, UCMJ, 10 U.S.C. §§ 892, 928, 934.1 The general court-martial, composed of a military judge sitting alone, sentenced him to a bad-conduct discharge, 8 months of confinement, forfeiture of all pay and allowances, and reduction to E-1. The convening authority limited the forfeiture of all pay and allowances to the time period Appellant was serving confinement, but otherwise approved the sentence as adjudged.

On appeal, Appellant contends that his convictions for assault consummated by a battery are factually insufficient in light of our superior court's decision in *United States v. Gutierrez*, 74 M.J. 61, 68 (C.A.A.F. 2015). He also argues that his convictions for willful dereliction of duty related to his failing to follow a safe-sex order directing him to inform sexual partners of his HIV-positive status and to use barrier protection during sex should be overturned as the order is overbroad and void for vagueness.

. . .

Appellant was originally charged with two specifications of assault by means likely to produce death or grievous bodily harm for engaging in sexual activity without disclosing his HIV-positive status; however, Appellant pled guilty to the lesser included offense of assault consummated by a battery. The first specification alleged that Appellant engaged in unprotected oral sex with divers [*sic*] sexual partners without disclosing his HIV-positive status. During his providence inquiry, Appellant explained he had unprotected oral sex with divers sexual partners in both Las Vegas, Nevada, and Columbia, South Carolina; and he did not tell any of them that he was HIV positive.

When the military judge specifically asked Appellant if he agreed that he engaged in a battery with the unlawful application of force, Appellant responded, "Yes, since they would not have consented if they knew my status. I now understand that constitutes force."

The second specification addressed the assaults consummated by a battery committed by Appellant when he engaged in protected anal sexual intercourse with divers sexual partners without informing them of his HIV-positive status. Appellant explained he used a condom when he engaged in anal sex with another male at the Las Vegas bathhouse. Appellant admitted he also had protected anal sex with men at each of the South Carolina hotel parties. He did not inform any of these partners that he was HIV positive. Appellant again admitted that his sexual activity with these men amounted to bodily harm because he *[footnote omitted]* did not tell them he was HIV positive and, that by not telling them, his bodily contact with them was without their knowing consent.

. . .

On appeal, we now consider the implication that if his partners had been HIV positive they would have consented. However, we find this bare speculation—without any support in the record—does not amount to a "substantial basis" to have us question the providence of Appellant's guilty plea. . . . Accordingly, we find no "substantial basis" to question the military judge's acceptance of Appellant's guilty plea. The findings of guilty for both specifications and the charge for assault consummated by a battery are affirmed.

. . .

Constitutional Challenge to the Safe-Sex Order
Appellant argues that his convictions for willful dereliction of duty for failing to obey his safe-sex orders should be overturned because the underlying safe-sex orders are unconstitutionally overbroad and void for vagueness.

. . .

Appellant *[also]* argues that his activity falls within the protected liberty interest identified by the Supreme Court in *Lawrence v. Texas*, 539 U.S. 558 (2003).

. . .

Appellant also makes a brief argument that the order is void for vagueness. . . . Appellant does not challenge the sufficiency of his plea and does not explain how he can providently plead guilty to a willful dereliction of a duty that is so vague as to be unconstitutional. Appellant admitted he had a duty, he knew of the duty, and he failed to perform that duty. He never indicated he had any problems understanding the order that created the duty. Appellant had actual knowledge of the order that imposed the duty and fair notice as to its requirements. "The guilty plea process within the military justice system thus ensures that an appellant has notice of the offense of which he may be convicted and all elements thereof before his plea is accepted and, moreover, protects him against double jeopardy." *United States v. Ballan*, 71 M.J. 28, 35 (C.A.A.F. 2012). Appellant's pleas were provident and the order was not void for vagueness.

Conclusion

The approved findings and the sentence are correct in law and fact, and no error materially prejudicial to the substantial rights of the appellant occurred.

Source: *United States v. Staff Sergeant Adolphus A. Young III*, United States Air Force ACM 38761 24 March 2016.

Sexually Transmitted Disease Surveillance 2015 (2016)

The U.S. Department of Health and Human Services publishes an annual report on the incidence and prevalence of sexually transmitted diseases (STDs) in the United States. The publication is intended as "a reference document for policy makers, program *managers, health planners, researchers, and others who are concerned with the public health implications of these diseases." The 2015 report contained some warnings about an uptick in the number of STD cases being reported, a comment reflected in the Foreword to the report, as cited here. (Triple asterisks [***] denote the omission of citations.)*

Sexually transmitted diseases (STDs) have long been an underestimated opponent in the public health battle. A 1997 Institute of Medicine (IOM) report described STDs as, "hidden epidemics of tremendous health and economic consequence in the United States," and stated that the "scope, impact, and consequences of STDs are underrecognized by the public and healthcare professionals."*** Since well before this report was published, and nearly two decades later, those facts remain unchanged.

It is estimated that there are 20 million new STDs in the U.S. each year, and half of these are among young people ages 15 to 24 years. Across the nation, at any given time, there are more than 110 million total (new and existing) infections. *** These infections can lead to long-term health consequences, such as infertility; they can facilitate HIV transmission; and they have stigmatized entire subgroups of Americans.

Yet not that long ago, gonorrhea rates were at historic lows, syphilis was close to elimination, and we were able to point to advances in STD prevention, such as better chlamydia diagnostic tests and more screening, contributing to increases in detection and treatment of chlamydial infections. That progress has since unraveled. The number of reported syphilis cases is climbing after being largely on the decline since 1941, and gonorrhea rates are now increasing. This is especially concerning given that we are slowly running out of treatment options to cure *Neisseria gonorrhoeae*. Many young women continue to have undiagnosed chlamydial infections, putting them at risk for infertility.

Beyond the impact on an individual's health, STDs are also an economic drain on the U.S. healthcare system. Data suggest the direct cost of treating STDs in the U.S. is nearly $16 billion annually. *** STD public health programs are increasingly facing challenges and barriers in achieving their mission. In 2012, 52% of state and local STD programs experienced budget cuts. This amounts to reductions in clinic hours, contact tracing, and screening for common STDs. CDC estimates that 21 local health department STD clinics closed that year. It is imperative that federal, state, and local programs employ strategies that maximize long-term population impact by reducing STD incidence and promoting sexual, reproductive, maternal, and infant health. The resurgence of syphilis, and particularly congenital syphilis, is not an arbitrary event, but rather a symptom of a deteriorating public health infrastructure and lack of access to health care. It is exposing hidden, fragile populations in need that are not getting the health care and preventive services they deserve. This points to our need for public health and health care action for each of the cases in this report, as they represent real people, not just numbers. We also need to modernize surveillance to move beyond counting only those cases in persons who have access to diagnosis and treatment, to develop innovative strategies to understand the burden of disease in those who may not access care, and to improve our surveillance systems to collect the information needed to target prevention activities. Further, it will be important for us to measure and monitor the adverse health consequences of STDs, such as ocular and neurosyphilis, pelvic inflammatory disease, ectopic pregnancy, infertility, HIV, congenital syphilis, and neonatal herpes.

It is my hope that a decade from now, we will be reporting on progress, instead of more health inequity in our society. This is our challenge and our call to effectively respond to the information shared in this report.

Gail Bolan, M.D.

Director, Division of STD Prevention

National Center for HIV/AIDS, Viral Hepatitis, STD, and

TB Prevention
U.S. Centers for Disease Control and Prevention

Source: Centers for Disease Control and Prevention. 2016. "Sexually Transmitted Disease Surveillance 2015." Atlanta: U.S. Department of Health and Human Services, v. Available online at https://www.cdc.gov/std/stats15/std-surveillance-2015-print.pdf. Accessed on February 7, 2017.

National Overview of Sexually Transmitted Diseases 2015 (2016)

The report cited above, "Sexually Transmitted Disease Surveillance 2015," also contains a summary of the statistics about syphilis, gonorrhea, and chlamydia that support Dr. Bolan's assessment of the status of STDs in the United States in 2015. That review makes the following points. (Triple asterisks [***] indicate the omission of certain citations.)

Chlamydia

In 2015, a total of 1,526,658 cases of *Chlamydia trachomatis* infection were reported to the CDC. This case count corresponds to a rate of 478.8 cases per 100,000 population, an increase of 5.9% compared with the rate in 2014. During 2014–2015, the rate of reported chlamydia cases among women increased 3.8% and the rate among men increased 10.5%. Following three years of decreases in rates during 2011–2014, the rate among women aged 15–19 years increased 1.5% during 2014–2015.

In 2015, the overall rate of chlamydial infection in the United States among women (645.5 cases per 100,000 females) based on reported cases was over two times the rate among men (305.2 cases per 100,000 males), reflecting the larger number of women screened for this infection. However, with the increased availability of urine testing and extragenital testing, men, including gay, bisexual, and other men who have sex with men (collectively referred to as MSM) are increasingly being tested for chlamydial infection. During 2011–2015, the chlamydia rate in men increased 20.0%, compared with a 0.3% increase in women during this period.

The facilities reporting chlamydial infections have changed over the last 10 years. In 2015, over 75% of chlamydia cases were reported from venues outside of STD clinics. Among women, only 4.5% of chlamydia cases were reported through an STD clinic and about a third of cases were reported from private physicians/health maintenance organizations.

Rates of reported chlamydia varied among different racial and ethnic minority populations. In 2015, the rate of chlamydia among Blacks was 5.9 times the rate among Whites, and the rate among American Indians/Alaska Natives was 3.8 times the rate among Whites.

Gonorrhea

In 2009, the national rate of reported gonorrhea cases reached an historic low of 98.1 cases per 100,000 population. However, during 2009–2012, the rate increased slightly each year to 106.7 cases per 100,000 population in 2012 and then increased again during 2013–2015. In 2015, 395,216 gonorrhea cases were reported for a rate of 123.9 cases per 100,000 population, an increase of 12.8% from 2014.

During 2014–2015 the rate of reported gonorrhea increased 18.3% among men and 6.8% among women. Gonorrhea rates among both men and women increased in every region of the United States, with largest increases in the West and the South. The magnitude of the increase among males suggest [*sic*] either increased transmission or increased case ascertainment (e.g., through increased extra-genital screening) among MSM or both.

In 2015, the rate of reported gonorrhea cases remained highest among Blacks (424.9 cases per 100,000 population) and among American Indians/Alaska Natives (192.8 cases per 100,000 population). While rates of gonorrhea declined 4.0%

among Blacks during 2011–2015, rates increased among all other racial and ethnic groups, including a 71.3% increase among American Indians/Alaska Natives.

Antimicrobial resistance remains an important consideration in the treatment of gonorrhea. With increased resistance to the fluoroquinolones and declining susceptibility to cefixime, dual therapy with ceftriaxone and azithromycin is now the only CDC recommended treatment for gonorrhea. ***

In 2015, the percentage of isolates with elevated minimum inhibitory concentrations (MICs) of cefixime and ceftriaxone remained low (0.5% and 0.3%, respectively). During 2013–2015, the percentage of isolates with reduced azithromycin susceptibility increased from 0.6% to 2.6%. Continued monitoring of susceptibility patterns to these antibiotics is critical.

Syphilis

In 2000 and 2001, the national rate of reported primary and secondary (P&S) syphilis cases was 2.1 cases per 100,000 population, the lowest rate since reporting began in 1941. However, the P&S syphilis rate has increased almost every year since 2001. In 2015, a total of 23,872 P&S syphilis cases were reported, and the national P&S syphilis rate increased to 7.5 cases per 100,000 population, a 19.0% increase from 2014.

During 2014–2015, the P&S syphilis rate increased both among men (18.1%) and women (27.3%) and rates increased among both sexes in every region of the country. Nationally, P&S syphilis rates increased in every 5-year age group among those aged 15–64 years and in every racial and ethnic group except for American Indians/Alaska Natives during 2014–2015.

During 2000–2015, the rise in the P&S syphilis rate was primarily attributable to increased cases among men and, specifically, among MSM. In 2015, men accounted for over 90% of all cases of P&S syphilis. Of those male cases for whom sex of sex partner was known, 81.7% were MSM. Reported cases of P&S syphilis continued to be characterized by a high rate of HIV co-infection, particularly among MSM. In the 31 states able to classify at least 70.0% of reported P&S syphilis cases as MSM, men who have sex with women (MSW), or women and at least 70.0% of reported cases as HIV-positive or HIV negative, 49.8% of MSM with P&S syphilis were also reported as HIV-positive compared with 10.0% of cases among MSW and 3.9% of cases among women.

The 2013 rate of congenital syphilis (9.2 cases per 100,000 live births) marked the first increase in congenital syphilis since 2008. During 2013–2014, the rate increased 27.2% and during 2014–2015 increased 6.0%, primarily attributable to an increase in the West. There were 487 cases of congenital syphilis reported in 2015 compared with 461 in 2014. Rates of congenital syphilis were highest among Blacks (35.2 cases per 100,000 live births), followed by Hispanics (15.5 cases per 100,000 live births) and American Indians/Alaska Natives (10.3 cases per 100,000 live births).

Source: Centers for Disease Control and Prevention. 2016. "Sexually Transmitted Disease Surveillance 2015." Atlanta: U.S. Department of Health and Human Services, 1–2. Available online at https://www.cdc.gov/std/stats15/std-surveillance-2015-print.pdf. Accessed on February 7, 2017.

Federal Legislation (as of 2017)

The U.S. Congress has passed relatively little legislation concerning STIs. The two major exceptions to that statement are an act dealing with the intentional or intentional transmission of the HIV virus between two individuals and federal assistance for STI prevention and treatment programs.

Payment of Cost of Testing for Sexually Transmitted Diseases (1994)

Although the title of this act refers to STIs, its content focuses exclusively on the HIV virus. It specifies the legal responsibilities of an individual who has committed a sexual act and may be infected with that virus.

§14011. Payment of cost of testing for sexually transmitted diseases

(a) Omitted

(b) Limited testing of defendants

    (1) Court order

        The victim of an offense of the type referred to in subsection (a) 1 of this section may obtain an order in the district court of the United States for the district in which charges are brought against the defendant charged with the offense, after notice to the defendant and an opportunity to be heard, requiring that the defendant be tested for the presence of the etiologic agent for acquired immune deficiency syndrome, and that the results of the test be communicated to the victim and the defendant. Any test result of the defendant given to the victim or the defendant must be accompanied by appropriate counseling.

    (2) Showing required

        To obtain an order under paragraph (1), the victim must demonstrate that—

        (A) the defendant has been charged with the offense in a State or Federal court, and if the defendant has been arrested without a warrant, a probable cause determination has been made;

        (B) the test for the etiologic agent for acquired immune deficiency syndrome is requested by the victim after appropriate counseling; and

        (C) the test would provide information necessary for the health of the victim of the alleged offense and the court determines that the alleged conduct of the defendant created a risk of transmission, as determined by the Centers for Disease Control, of the etiologic agent for acquired immune deficiency syndrome to the victim.

(3) Follow-up testing

The court may order follow-up tests and counseling under paragraph (1) if the initial test was negative. Such follow-up tests and counseling shall be performed at the request of the victim on dates that occur six months and twelve months following the initial test.

(4) Termination of testing requirements

An order for follow-up testing under paragraph (3) shall be terminated if the person obtains an acquittal on, or dismissal of, all charges of the type referred to in subsection (a) 1 of this section.

(5) Confidentiality of test

The results of any test ordered under this subsection shall be disclosed only to the victim or, where the court deems appropriate, to the parent or legal guardian of the victim, and to the person tested. The victim may disclose the test results only to any medical professional, counselor, family member or sexual partner(s) the victim may have had since the attack. Any such individual to whom the test results are disclosed by the victim shall maintain the confidentiality of such information.

(6) Disclosure of test results

The court shall issue an order to prohibit the disclosure by the victim of the results of any test performed under this subsection to anyone other than those mentioned in paragraph (5). The contents of the court proceedings and test results pursuant to this section shall be sealed. The results of such test performed on the defendant under this section shall not be used as evidence in any criminal trial.

(7) Contempt for disclosure

Any person who discloses the results of a test in violation of this subsection may be held in contempt of court.

(c) Penalties for intentional transmission of HIV

Not later than 6 months after September 13, 1994, the United States Sentencing Commission shall conduct a study and prepare and submit to the committees on the Judiciary of the Senate and the House of Representatives a report concerning recommendations for the revision of sentencing guidelines that relate to offenses in which an HIV infected individual engages in sexual activity if the individual knows that he or she is infected with HIV and intends, through such sexual activity, to expose another to HIV.

Source: 42 U.S. Code § 14011.

Sexually Transmitted Diseases; Prevention and Control Projects and Programs (2017)

Over a period of more than 40 years, the U.S. Congress has provided federal funding for a variety of research, educational, and other activities aimed at the prevention and treatment of STIs. The current provision for such activities is included in Section 247c of Title 42 of the U.S. Code.

42 U.S. Code § 247c—Sexually transmitted diseases; prevention and control projects and programs

(a) Technical assistance to public and nonprofit private entities and scientific institutions

The Secretary may provide technical assistance to appropriate public and nonprofit private entities and to scientific institutions for their research in, and training and public health programs for, the prevention and control of sexually transmitted diseases.

(b) Research, demonstration, and public information and education projects

The Secretary may make grants to States, political subdivisions of States, and any other public and nonprofit private entity for—

(1) research into the prevention and control of sexually transmitted diseases;

(2) demonstration projects for the prevention and control of sexually transmitted diseases;

(3) public information and education programs for the prevention and control of such diseases; and

(4) education, training, and clinical skills improvement activities in the prevention and control of such diseases for health professionals (including allied health personnel).

(c) Project grants to States

The Secretary is also authorized to make project grants to States and, in consultation with the State health authority, to political subdivisions of States, for—

(1) sexually transmitted diseases surveillance activities, including the reporting, screening, and followup of diagnostic tests for, and diagnosed cases of, sexually transmitted diseases;

(2) casefinding and case followup activities respecting sexually transmitted diseases, including contact tracing of infectious cases of sexually transmitted diseases and routine testing, including laboratory tests and followup systems;

(3) interstate epidemiologic referral and followup activities respecting sexually transmitted diseases; and

(4) such special studies or demonstrations to evaluate or test sexually transmitted diseases prevention and control strategies and activities as may be prescribed by the Secretary.

(d) Grants for innovative, interdisciplinary approaches

The Secretary may make grants to States and political subdivisions of States for the development, implementation, and evaluation of innovative, interdisciplinary approaches to the prevention and control of sexually transmitted diseases.

(e) Authorization of appropriations; terms and conditions; payments; recordkeeping; audit; grant reduction; information disclosure

[This section provides details about the manner in which grants are to be made.]

(5)   All information obtained in connection with the examination, care, or treatment of any individual under any program which is being carried out with a grant made under this section shall not, without such individual's consent, be disclosed except as may be necessary to provide service to him or as may be required by a law of a state or political subdivision of a State. Information derived from any such program may be disclosed—

(A)   in summary, statistical, or other form; or

(B)   for clinical or research purposes;

but only if the identity of the individuals diagnosed or provided care or treatment under such program is not disclosed.

(f) Consent of individuals

Nothing in this section shall be construed to require any State or any political subdivision of a State to have a sexually transmitted diseases program which would require any person, who objects to any treatment provided under such a program, to be treated under such a program.

Source: 42 U.S. Code § 247c.

State Laws (as of 2017)

Every state in the Union has one or more (often, many more) laws dealing with STIs. These laws cover a wide range of topics associated with STIs in greater or lesser detail. A superb summary of those laws can be found at https://www.cdc.gov/std/program/final-std-statutesall-states-5june-2014.pdf. The following sections list some of the most common areas covered by state laws, with one example from state statutes in each case.

Reportable Disease

Every state has some type of statute that requires healthcare workers and others who may deal with infected individuals to submit a formal report about every case of STI with which they come into contact.

Example: Wyoming: 35-4-132. **Report required of health care providers, facilities and laboratories; notification; confidentiality of information.**

(a) A physician or other health care provider diagnosing or treating a case of sexually transmitted disease, the administrator of a hospital, dispensary, charitable or penal institution or any other health care facility in which there is a case of sexually transmitted disease and the administrator or operator of a laboratory performing a positive laboratory test for sexually transmitted disease shall report the diagnosis, case or positive test results to both the department of health and the appropriate health officer in a form and manner directed by the department. Health care providers and facilities shall cooperate with and assist the department and health officers in preventing the spread of sexually transmitted disease.

(b) The department of health shall compile the number of reported cases within the state.

(c) Any physician or other health care provider and any administrator or operator of a health care facility or laboratory reporting a diagnosis, case or positive test result pursuant to subsection (a) of this section shall notify any health care professional and health care employee reasonably expected to be at risk of exposure to a dangerous or life threatening sexually transmitted disease and involved in the supervision, care and treatment of an individual infected or reasonably suspected of being infected with a dangerous or life threatening sexually transmitted disease.

(d) Information and records relating to a known or suspected case of sexually transmitted disease which has been reported, acquired and maintained under W.S. 35 4 130 through 35 4 134 are confidential and except as otherwise required by law, shall not be disclosed unless the disclosure is:

(i)   For statistical purposes, provided that the identity of the individual with the known or suspected case is protected;

(ii) Necessary for the administration and enforcement of W.S. 35 4 130 through 35 4 134 and department rules and regulations related to the control and treatment of sexually transmitted diseases;

(iii) Made with the written consent of the individual identified within the information or records; or

(iv) For notification of health care professionals and health care employees pursuant to subsection (c) of this section as necessary to protect life and health.

Confidentiality

Most states include some provision for ensuring that all medical records regarding STIs are kept private.

Example: New Mexico: 24-1-9.4. **Sexually transmitted diseases; confidentiality.**

Except as provided in Section 24-1-9.2 NMSA 1978, no person or the person's agents or employees who require or administer a test for sexually transmitted diseases shall disclose the identity of any person upon whom a test is performed or the result of such a test in a manner that permits identification of the subject of the test, except to the following persons:

A. the subject of the test or the subject's legally authorized representative, guardian or legal custodian;

B. any person designated in a legally effective release of the test results executed prior to or after the test by the subject of the test or the subject's legally authorized representative;

C. an authorized agent, a credentialed or privileged physician or employee of a health facility or health care provider if the health care facility or health care provider itself is authorized to obtain the test results, the agent or employee provides patient care or handles or processes specimens of body fluids or tissues and the agent or employee has a need to know such information;

D. the department of health and the centers for disease control and prevention of the United States public health service in accordance with reporting requirements for a diagnosed case of a sexually transmitted disease;

E. a health facility or health care provider that procures, processes, distributes or uses:

(1) a human body part from a deceased person, with respect to medical information regarding that person;

(2) semen for the purpose of artificial insemination;

(3) blood or blood products for transfusion or injection; or

(4) human body parts for transplant with respect to medical information regarding the donor or recipient;

F. health facility staff committees or accreditation or over-sight review organizations that are conducting program monitoring, program evaluation or service reviews, as long as any identity remains confidential;

G. authorized medical or epidemiological researchers who may not further disclose any identifying characteristics or information; and

H. for purposes of application or reapplication for insurance coverage, an insurer or reinsurer upon whose request the test was performed.

STI Education

Another popular component of state laws dealing with STI is some type of requirement that the state and/or local communities provide some form of education about STIs.

Example: Minnesota 121A.23. **Programs to Prevent and Reduce the Risks of Sexually Transmitted Infections and Diseases.**

Subdivision 1. Sexually transmitted infections and diseases program. The commissioner of education, in consultation with the commissioner of health, shall assist districts in developing and implementing a program to prevent and reduce the risk of sexually transmitted infections and diseases, including but not exclusive to human immune deficiency virus and human papilloma virus. Each district must have a program that includes at least:

(1) planning materials, guidelines, and other technically accurate and updated information;

(2) a comprehensive, technically accurate, and updated curriculum that includes helping students to abstain from sexual activity until marriage;

(3) cooperation and coordination among districts and SCs;

(4) a targeting of adolescents, especially those who may be at high risk of contracting sexually transmitted infections and diseases, for prevention efforts;

(5) involvement of parents and other community members;

(6) in-service training for appropriate district staff and school board members;

(7) collaboration with state agencies and organizations having a sexually transmitted infection and disease prevention or sexually transmitted infection and disease risk reduction program;

(8) collaboration with local community health services, agencies and organizations having a sexually transmitted infection and disease prevention or sexually transmitted infection and disease risk reduction program; and

(9) participation by state and local student organizations.

The department may provide assistance at a neutral site to a nonpublic school participating in a district's program. District programs must not conflict with the health and wellness curriculum developed under Laws 1987, chapter 398, article 5, section 2, subdivision 7.

If a district fails to develop and implement a program to prevent and reduce the risk of sexually transmitted infection and disease, the department must assist the service cooperative in the region serving that district to develop or implement the program.

Subd. 2. Funding sources. Districts may accept funds for sexually transmitted infection and disease prevention programs developed and implemented under this section from public and private sources including public health funds and foundations, department professional development funds, federal block grants or other federal or state grants.

Partner Notification

Many states provide a system for notifying spouses or partners of a person infected with an STI, either as a voluntary or required action.

Example: Maine Title 22 §1242. **Expedited partner therapy.**

Notwithstanding any other provision of law, a health care professional who makes a clinical diagnosis of a sexually transmitted disease may provide expedited partner therapy for the treatment of the sexually transmitted disease if in the judgment of the health care professional the sexual partner is unlikely or unable to present for comprehensive health care, including evaluation, testing and treatment for sexually transmitted diseases. Expedited partner therapy is limited to a sexual partner who may have been exposed to a sexually transmitted disease within the previous 60 days and who is able to be contacted by the patient.

1. Counseling. A health care professional who provides expedited partner therapy shall provide counseling for the patient, including advice that all women and symptomatic persons, and in particular women with symptoms suggestive of pelvic inflammatory disease, are encouraged to seek medical attention. The health care professional shall also provide written materials provided by the department to be given by the patient to the sexual partner that include at a minimum the following:

   A. A warning that a woman who is pregnant or might be pregnant should not take certain antibiotics and should immediately contact a health care professional for an examination;

   B. Information about the antibiotic and dosage provided or prescribed; clear and explicit allergy and side effect warnings, including a warning that a sexual partner who has a history of allergy to the antibiotic or the pharmaceutical class of antibiotic should not take the antibiotic and should be immediately examined by a health care professional;

   C. Information about the treatment and prevention of sexually transmitted diseases;

   D. The requirement of abstinence until a period of time after treatment to prevent infecting others;

E. Notification of the importance of the sexual partner's receiving examination and testing for the human immunodeficiency virus and other sexually transmitted diseases and information regarding available resources;

F. Notification of the risk to the sexual partner, others and the public health if the sexually transmitted disease is not completely and successfully treated;

G. The responsibility of the sexual partner to inform that person's sexual partners of the risk of sexually transmitted disease and the importance of prompt examination and treatment;

H. Advice to all women and symptomatic persons, and in particular women with symptoms suggestive of pelvic inflammatory disease, to seek medical attention; and

I. Information other than the information under paragraphs A to H as determined necessary by the department.

2. Department to develop and disseminate materials. Taking into account the recommendations of the federal Department of Health and Human Services, Centers for Disease Control and Prevention and other nationally recognized medical authorities, the department shall provide information and technical assistance as appropriate to health care professionals who provide expedited partner therapy. The department shall develop and disseminate in electronic and other formats the following written materials:

A. Informational materials for sexual partners, as described in subsection 1;

B. Informational materials for persons who are repeatedly diagnosed with sexually transmitted diseases; and

C. Guidance for health care professionals on the safe and effective provision of expedited partner therapy. The department may offer educational programs about expedited partner therapy for health care professionals and pharmacists licensed under the Maine Pharmacy Act.

3. Immunity for health care professional. A health care professional who provides expedited partner therapy in good faith without fee or compensation under this section and provides counseling and written materials as required in subsection 1 is not subject to civil or professional liability in connection with the provision of the therapy, counseling and materials, except in the case of willful and wanton misconduct. A health care professional is not subject to civil or professional liability for choosing not to provide expedited partner therapy.

4. Immunity for pharmacist or pharmacy. A pharmacist or pharmacy is not subject to civil or professional liability for choosing not to fill a prescription that would cause that pharmacist or pharmacy to violate any provision of the Maine Pharmacy Act 1.

Testing of Prisoners
Many states require STI testing of certain populations of individuals, perhaps the most common of which includes those who have been incarcerated in jails and prisons.

Example: South Carolina 44-29-100. **Examination and treatment of prisoners for sexually transmitted disease; isolation and treatment after serving sentence.**

Any person who is confined or imprisoned in any state, county, or city prison of this State may be examined and treated for a sexually transmitted disease by the health authorities or their deputies. The state, county, and municipal boards of health may take over a portion of any state, county, or city prison for use as a board of health hospital. Persons who are confined or imprisoned and who are suffering with a sexually transmitted disease at the time of expiration of their terms of imprisonment must be isolated and treated at public expense as provided in Section 44-29-90 until, in the judgment of the local health officer, the prisoner may be medically discharged. In lieu of isolation, the person, in the discretion of the board of health, may be required to report for treatment to a licensed physician or submit for treatment provided at public expense by the Department of Health and Environmental Control as provided in Section 44-29-90.

Anyone Convicted (or Accused) of a Sexual Assault

Another category of individuals who may be required to have blood test for an STI are individuals who have been convicted of sexual assault or, much less commonly, anyone who has been accused of such an assault, whether he or she has been convicted of the crime or not.

Example: Pennsylvania Title 35 § 521.8. **Venereal disease.**

(a) Any person taken into custody and charged with any crime involving lewd conduct or a sex offense, or any person to whom the jurisdiction of a juvenile court attaches, may be examined for a venereal disease by a qualified physician appointed by the department or by the local board or department of health or appointed by the court having jurisdiction over the person so charged.

(b) Any person convicted of a crime or pending trial, who is confined in or committed to any State or local penal institution, reformatory or any other house of correction or detention, may be examined for venereal disease by a qualified physician appointed by the department or by the local board or department of health or by the attending physician of the institution, if any.

Reasonable Cause

There are times when an officer of the law has reason to believe that a particular individual may have an STI and may also be engaging in activities that are likely to result in transmission of that disease. In some states, laws exist that allow such officers of the law to take action against those suspected of being infected.

Example: Wisconsin. 252.11.(2) **Sexually transmitted disease**.

An officer of the department or a local health officer having knowledge of any reported or reasonably suspected case or contact of a sexually transmitted disease for which no appropriate treatment is being administered, or of an actual contact of a reported case or potential contact of a reasonably suspected case, shall investigate or cause the case or contact to be investigated as necessary. If, following a request of an officer of the department or a local health officer, a person reasonably suspected of being infected with a sexually transmitted disease refuses or neglects examination by a physician, physician assistant, or advanced practice nurse prescriber or treatment, an officer of the department or a local health officer may proceed to have the person committed under sub. (5) to an institution or system of care for examination, treatment, or observation.

Quarantine

Among the most severe legal provisions dealing with STIs are those that permit isolation, imprisonment, or other actions against a person who has an STI.

Example: Mississippi. 41-23-27. **Infectious sexually transmitted diseases**.

The state board of health shall have full power to isolate, quarantine or otherwise confine, intern, and treat such person afflicted with such infectious sexually transmitted disease for such time and under such restrictions as may seem proper. Said board shall have full power to pass all such rules and regulations as to the isolation, quarantine, confinement, internment and treatment as may be needful.

Any person knowingly violating any rule or regulation promulgated by the state board of health, under the authority of this section, shall be deemed guilty of a misdemeanor and upon conviction shall be punished by fine or imprisonment or both.

Human Papillomavirus Vaccine

Although more than half of the states have considered requiring vaccination with the human papillomavirus vaccine as a condition for school entrance, only one state, Virginia, and the District of Columbia have actually adopted such as law.

Virginia law: **An Act to amend and reenact § 32.1-46 of the Code of Virginia, relating to requiring the human papillomavirus vaccine (32.1-46).**

A. The parent, guardian or person standing in loco parentis of each child within this Commonwealth shall cause such child to be immunized. . .

The required immunizations for attendance at a public or private elementary, middle or secondary school, child care center, nursery school, family day care home or developmental center shall be. . .

12. Three doses of properly spaced human papillomavirus (HPV) vaccine for females. The first dose shall be administered before the child enters the sixth grade.

While most states have not enacted requirements for HPV vaccinations, many have mandated a variety of other actions to encourage better understanding of the disease and the value of the vaccine. These actions include educational campaigns, free vaccination programs, and requirements that vaccinations be covered by health insurance programs in the state.

Example: Missouri: 167.182. **HPV informational brochure, contents.**

167.182. 1. The department of health and senior services shall develop an informational brochure relating to the connection between human papillomavirus and cervical cancer, and that an immunization against the human papillomavirus infection is available. The department shall make the brochure available on its website and shall notify each public school district in this state of the availability of the brochure to be printed and included or referred to in any other printed material to be provided directly to parents as the school district deems appropriate. However, materials made available pursuant to this section may only be distributed to parents directly and not distributed to students as material to be given to parents. Such information in the brochure shall include:

(1) The risk factors for developing cervical cancer, the symptoms of the disease, how it may be diagnosed, and its possible consequences if untreated;

(2) The connection between human papillomavirus and cervical cancer, how human papillomavirus is transmitted, how transmission may be prevented, including abstinence as the best way to prevent sexually transmitted diseases, and the relative risk of contracting human papillomavirus for primary and secondary school students;

(3) The latest scientific information on the immunization against human papillomavirus infection and the immunization's effectiveness against causes of cervical cancer;

(4) That a pap smear is still critical for the detection of precancerous changes in the cervix to allow for treatment before cervical cancer develops; and

(5) A statement that any questions or concerns regarding immunizing the child against human papillomavirus could be answered by contacting the family's health care provider.

Source: Official statutes of states listed.

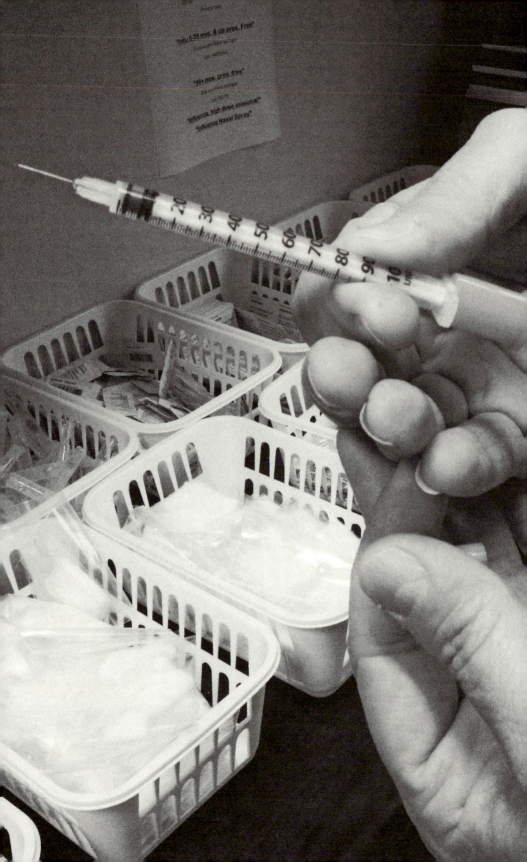

Introduction

Sexually transmitted infections (STIs) is a topic of significant interest to both professionals in the field and the average man or woman, boy or girl. Untold numbers of books, articles, book chapters, reports, and web pages have been devoted to a discussion of one or more aspects of this subject. This bibliography can provide no more than a sampling of some of the most recent of these items, as well as some publications of historical interest. In some cases, an item has appeared both in print and on the Internet, in which case it is so designated in the print listing.

Books

Arrizabalaga, Jon, John Henderson, and Roger French. 1997. *The Great Pox: The French Disease in Renaissance Europe*. New Haven, CT: Yale University Press.

> This book is particularly valuable, not only because it describes the early decades following the appearance of syphilis in Europe, but also because it discusses the social,

---

A public health nurse for eastern Indiana's Fayette County, holds one of the syringes provided to intravenous drug users taking part in the county's state-approved needle exchange program, The cash-strapped rural county was facing a hepatitis C outbreak among IV drug users. It was one of the Indiana counties to win state approval for the programs that provide those users with clean needles to reduce needle-sharing as a way to stop the spread of HIV, hepatitis C and other diseases. (AP Photo/Rick Callahan)

political, religious, and other responses to the spread of the disease. This discussion has considerable significance to issues relating to the worldwide spread of STIs in today's world. In this respect, also see Knell 2004, under Internet, below.

Bachmann, Laura Hinkle. 2017. *Sexually Transmitted Infections in HIV-infected Adults and Special Populations: A Clinical Guide.* Berlin; New York: Springer Verlag.
  The papers in this collection deal with many aspect of issues surrounding the coinfection of HIV with a variety of STIs.

Berco, Cristian. 2016. *From Body to Community: Venereal Disease and Society in Baroque Spain.* Toronto, Buffalo: University of Toronto Press.
  This book provides a fascinating look at the way STIs were regarded during a very specific place and period in history: baroque Spain in the first half of the 17th century.

Brandt, Allan M. 1987. *No Magic Bullet: A Social History of Venereal Disease in the United States since 1880.* New York: Oxford University Press.
  This book traces the history of American attitudes toward and behaviors regarding STIs, beginning with Victorian hysteria about syphilis and continuing to modern-day concerns about acquired immune deficiency syndrome (AIDS) and other STIs. The author shows how various parts of society, such as the medical, military, and the public health community, have responded to the issue of STIs. He notes that, in general, Americans' attitudes toward STIs as being sinful or "earned" by those who develop the diseases have impeded efforts to develop drugs that would effectively halt the spread of infection.

Brunette, Gary W., et al. 2016. *CDC Health Information for International Travel.* New York: Oxford University Press. Available online at https://global.oup.com/academic/product/cdc-health-information-for-international-travel-2016-9780199379156? q=cdc%202016&lang=en&cc=us#. Accessed on April 4, 2017.

This biennial publication is one of the most reliable references on the types of diseases that can be contracted while traveling outside the United States. The extensive list of diseases covered includes a number of STIs, both well known and less well known.

Collins, Beverly. 2015. *Updated Researches in Chlamydia.* Jersey City, NJ: Foster Academics.

This book attempts to bring the reader up-do-date on all aspects of the diagnosis, biology, prevention, and treatment of chlamydia.

Davidson, Roger, and Lesley A. Hall. 2011. *Sex, Sin and Suffering: Venereal Disease and European Society since 1870.* London: Routledge.

The 14 essays that make up this book deal with accounts of very specific examples of the way STIs have been dealt with in a variety of European nations, such as syphilis and prostitution in 19th-century France, Swedish social policy on STIs in the early 20th century, and attitudes toward STIs in revolutionary Russia.

Dunbar, Raden. 2014. *The Secrets of the Anzacs: The Untold Story of Venereal Disease in the Australian Army, 1914–1919.* Melbourne: Scribe.

The author tells an intriguing story about an STI epidemic that developed within the Australian–New Zealand armed forces during World War I.

Eaton, Lisa A., and Seth C. Kalichman, eds. 2014. *Biomedical Advances in HIV Prevention: Social and Behavioral Perspectives.* New York: Springer.

This volume summarizes recent developments in medical and social methods for reducing the transmission of the

HIV virus, with chapters on topics such as pre-exposure prophylaxis (PrEP) and its efficacy, mental health and substance abuse among HIV-infected individuals, and implementing HIV prevention technologies in three specific nations—Ecuador, Thailand, and Uganda.

Gray, Fred D. 2013. *The Tuskegee Syphilis Study: The Real Story and Beyond.* Montgomery, AL: NewSouth Books.

The author was attorney for the men involved in the notorious Tuskegee syphilis study that ran from 1932 to 1972. He discusses the background of the study, the investigation that led to the lawsuit in which he was involved, and the events that led up to a presidential apology by Bill Clinton in 1997.

Grimes, Jill. 2016. *Seductive Delusions: How Everyday People Catch STIs.* Baltimore: Johns Hopkins University Press.

This book provides a "down-to-earth" description of major STIs, along with chapters on related issues, such as cervical cancer and date rape.

Grimes, Jill, Kristyn Fagerberg, and Lori Smith. 2014. *Sexually Transmitted Disease: An Encyclopedia of Diseases, Prevention, Treatment, and Issues.* Santa Barbara, CA: Greenwood Press.

This book provides an excellent introduction to and resource for basic concepts in the field of STIs.

Gross, Gerd, and Stephen K. Tyring. 2011. *Sexually Transmitted Infections and Sexually Transmitted Diseases.* Berlin: Springer.

This book covers a wide variety of topics related to STIs, including a history of STIs, the epidemiology of such diseases, sexual behavior and psychological aspects associated with STIs, detailed discussions of the most common varieties of infections, the status of STIs in various parts of the world, and some economic and political issues associated with STIs.

Handsfield, H. Hunter. 2011. *Color Atlas & Synopsis of Sexually Transmitted Diseases*, 3rd ed. New York: McGraw Hill.

This book is a well-illustrated review of bacterial and viral STIs along with a detailed description of signs and symptoms of the diseases discussed.

Handsfield, H. Hunter, et al. 2012. *Expedited Partner Therapy in the Management of Sexually Transmitted Diseases*. New York: Nova Science Publishers.

This short book provides the basic principles behind expedited partner therapy and outlines procedures for putting it into practice.

Holmes, King, et al., eds. 2008. *Sexually Transmitted Diseases*, 4th ed. New York: McGraw Hill Medical.

This book is one of the best known and most widely used books in the field of STIs with sections on the history, socioeconomic impact, and epidemiology of STIs; social and psychological aspects of sexuality; profiles of vulnerable populations; host immunity and molecular pathogenesis and STIs; sexually transmitted viral pathogens; sexually transmitted bacterial pathogens; overview of sexually transmitted disease (STD) care management; and nearly a dozen other topics.

Kamberg, Mary-Lane. 2016. *Chlamydia*. New York: Rosen Publishing.

This book is intended for young adults who are looking for a general introduction to the topic of chlamydia.

Katz, Ralph V., and Rueben C. Warren, eds. 2013. *The Search for the Legacy of the USPHS Syphilis Study at Tuskegee*. Lanham, MD: Lexington Books.

This collection of 14 papers dealing with the Tuskegee syphilis study of 1932–1972 deal with a number of issues relating to the study, including the ethical conduct of the study, "racial conspiracy and research," and the legacy of the study for science and ethics.

Khanna, Neena. 2012. *Illustrated Synopsis of Dermatology and Sexually Transmitted Diseases*, 4th ed. New Delhi: Elsevier.
This book provides a comprehensive overview of all known STIs along with a large number of color illustrations showing characteristic feature of each disease.

Kumar, Bhushan, and Somesh Gupta. 2012. *Sexually Transmitted Infections*, 2nd ed. New Delhi: Elsevier.
This book is a particularly good introduction to all aspects of STIs, with an introductory chapter that covers the history of the diseases in a concise but very useful format.

Lowry, Thomas Power. 2014. *Civil War Venereal Disease Hospitals*. Charleston, SC: Createspace.
Reports of deaths and injuries both on the battlefield and behind the scenes during the Civil War have been widely written and commented about. This book focuses on the special issue of STIs among participants in the war. The problem was serious enough that two hospitals during the time were reserved exclusively and entirely for treating STIs.

Moffat, Celia, and Joel Matyanga. 2014. *Pre-Exposure Prophylaxis for HIV Prevention: Truvada, a Pill for HIV Prevention*. Saarbruüken: LAP Lambert Academic Publishing.
This book provides a comprehensive and detailed introduction to the development and use of the first medication to be approved for the prevention of HIV infections.

Neilan, Anne M. 2016. "Sexually Transmitted Infections (STIs) in Adolescents." In Mark A. Goldstein, ed. *The MassGeneral Hospital for Children Adolescent Medicine Handbook*. New York: Springer, 207–236.
The author provides a general overview of the status of STIs in adolescents in the United States, noting that there

are five general principles to the prevention of such infections: education and counseling of patients at risk for STI; identification of asymptomatic patients with STI who are unlikely to seek treatment; effective diagnosis and treatment of STI; effective diagnosis and treatment of partners of patients with STI; and identification and immunization of patients at risk for vaccine preventable STI.

Orr, Tamara. 2016. *Gonorrhea*. New York: Rosen Publishing.
This book is intended for young adults as part of the publisher's Your Sexual Health series.

Passos, Mauro Romero Leal, ed. 2018. *Atlas of Sexually Transmitted Diseases Clinical Aspects and Differential Diagnosis*. Cham, Switzerland: Springer International Publishing.
This book provides detailed descriptions of all STIs with about 1,000 illustrations for identification of thediseases.

Rosenbaum, Julius. 1901. *The Plague of Lust, Being a History of Venereal Disease in Classical Antiquity*, 2 vols. Paris: Charles Carrington. Available online at https://archive.org/details/plagueoflustbein01rose and https://archive.org/details/plagueof lustbein02rose. Accessed on February 10, 2017.
This now outdated work provides a great deal of information, sometimes of dubious reliability, but often of considerable interest, about the existence of STIs in the ancient world.

Sanford, A. Christopher, Paul S. Pottinger, and Elaine C. Jong. 2017. *The Travel and Tropical Medicine Manual*. Edinburgh, New York: Elsevier.
Section 6 of this book deals with the STDs that one is likely to encounter in travels outside the United States, along with their characteristic features, prevention, and treatment.

Schlossberg, David, ed. 2015. *Clinical Infectious Disease*. Cambridge, UK: Cambridge University Press.

This book arranges a host of infectious disease by site of most common infection, such as head and neck, eye, skin and lymph nodes, and respiratory tract. An expert in each area describes the manifestations and treatment of all major STIs at the appropriate body location.

Sehgal, Virendra. 2013. *Donovanosis (Granuloma Inguinale)*, 2nd ed. New Delhi: Jaypee Brothers Medical Publishers.
This book provides one of the most complete descriptions of donovanosis currently available, with chapters on its epidemiological features, clinical presentation, laboratory diagnosis, and treatment options.

Shilts, Randy. 1987. *And the Band Played On*. New York: St. Martin's Press.
This book is an essential reading for anyone who is interested in the early social, political, and medical history of the AIDS epidemic.

Skolnik, Neil S., Amy Lynn Clouse, and Jo Ann Woodward, eds. 2013. *Sexually Transmitted Diseases: A Practical Guide for Primary Care*. Totowa, NJ: Humana Press.
This book provides good general introductions on a dozen major STIs, with an emphasis on methods of treatment for each condition.

Wilton, Leo, et al., eds. 2015. *Understanding HIV and STI Prevention for College Students*. New York; Oxfordshire, England: Routledge.
The papers that make up this book discuss topics such as methods of improving knowledge of STIs among the digital generation of students; popular culture and the improvement of sexual health practices; college women, sexual assault, and HIV/STI prevention; HIV and STI prevention among lesbian, gay, bisexual, and transgender students; religion, spirituality, and STI issues; and HIV and STI prevention in minority-serving institutions.

Wolny, Philip. 2015. *I Have an STD. Now What?* New York: Rosen Publishing.

This book is designed for teenagers. It provides a general introduction to the major types of STIs, what their symptoms are, and how they can be prevented and treated.

Zenilman, Jonathan M., and Mohsen Shahmanesh, eds. 2012. *Sexually Transmitted Infections: Diagnosis, Management, and Treatment.* Sudbury, MA: Jones & Bartlett Learning.

This book has separate chapters on 13 specific STIs along with more than 30 additional chapters on related issues, such as prevention counseling and condom use, partner notification and management care following rape and sexual assault, HIV counseling and testing, and sexually transmitted infections during pregnancy.

Articles

Some journals that specialize in articles on sexually transmitted infections are the following:

AIDS Patient Care and STDs. ISSN Print: 1087-2914; Online ISSN: 1557-7449

Indian Journal of Sexually Transmitted Diseases and AIDS. ISSN Print: 0253-7184; ISSN Online: 1998-3816

International Journal of STD & AIDS. ISSN Print: 0956–4624; ISSN Online: 1758–1052

Journal of Sexually Transmitted Diseases. ISSN Print: 2090-7893; ISSN Online: 2090-7958; DOI: 10.1155/1905

Sexually Transmitted Diseases. ISSN: 0148-5717

Sexually Transmitted Infections. ISSN Print: 1368-4973; ISSN Online: 1472-3263

Aeschlimann, John A., et al. 1954. "Paul Ehrlich Centennial." *Annals of the New York Academy of Science*, 59: 143–276.

The papers that make up this volume discuss Ehrlich's contributions to science in a number of fields and covering a number of topics such as staining techniques; chemotherapy of trypanosome, spirochetal, and bacterial infections; cancer research; and drug resistance.

Aspinall, Esther J., et al. 2014. "Are Needle and Syringe Programmes Associated with a Reduction in HIV Transmission among People Who Inject Drugs: A Systematic Review and Meta-Analysis." *International Journal of Epidemiology*, 43(1): 235-248.

The authors report on a meta-analysis of 12 studies on the effectiveness of needle exchange programs to change individuals' behaviors that may contribute to increased risk for HIV infections. They conclude that such programs should be thought of "as just one component of a programme of interventions to reduce both injecting risk and other types of HIV risk behaviour."

Barbee, Lindley A. 2014. "Preparing for an Era of Untreatable Gonorrhea." *Current Opinion in Infectious Diseases*, 27(3): 282-287. Available online at https://www.ncbi.nlm.nih.gov/pmc/articles/PMC4097387/. Accessed on April 1, 2017.

The author reviews the current state of untreatable gonorrhea and suggests some steps that can be taken to deal with the disease as treatment becomes more problematic. He recommends "screening for asymptomatic infections, maintaining culture capacity to monitor antimicrobial resistance, treating with ceftriaxone plus azithromycin, and ensuring that all sexual partners are treated."

Basta-Juzbašić, Aleksandra, and Romana Čeović. 2014. "Chancroid, Lymphogranuloma Venereum, Granuloma Inguinale, Genital Herpes Simplex Infection, and Molluscum Contagiosum." *Clinics in Dermatology*, 32(2): 290–298.

The authors provide detailed descriptions on four STIs, three of which are perhaps less well known and less common in the United States.

Bradshaw, Catriona S., and Jack D. Sobel. 2016. "Current Treatment of Bacterial Vaginosis—Limitations and Need for Innovation." *The Journal of Infectious Diseases*, 214(Suppl 1): S14-S20.

The authors remind readers of the limited options available for treating bacterial vaginosis and suggest some possible new approaches to the development of substances that can attack the causative agents of the disease.

Bulir, D. C., et al. 2016. "Immunization with Chlamydial Type III Secretion Antigens Reduces Vaginal Shedding and Prevents Fallopian Tube Pathology Following Live *C. Muridarum* Challenge Format. *Vaccine*, 34(34): 3979-3985.

This article reports on progress being made in the development of a vaccine for chlamydia strains. For a less technical explanation, see Alexander in the Internet section below.

Burg, Giovanni. 2012. "History of Sexually Transmitted Infections (STI)." *Giornale Italiano Di Dermatologia E Venereologia*, 147(4): 329-340.

This article provides a good general overview of current information about the primary events that have occurred in human understanding of the nature of STIs.

Chesson, Harrell W., et al. 2014. "Ciprofloxacin Resistance and Gonorrhea Incidence Rates in 17 Cities, United States, 1991–2006." *Emerging Infectious Diseases*, 20(4): 612-619. Available online at https://wwwnc.cdc.gov/eid/article/20/4/13-1288_article. Accessed on April 1, 2017.

The spread of nontreatable gonorrhea has begun to spread widely in the United States. This article provides some of the quantitative data that are available to confirm that spread.

Chow Eric P. F., et al. 2016. "Antiseptic Mouthwash against Pharyngeal *Neisseria Gonorrhoeae*: A Randomised Controlled Trial and an In Vitro Study." *Sexually Transmitted Infections*, 93: 88-93. Available online at http://sti.bmj.com/content/sextrans/93/2/88.full.pdf. Accessed on March 31, 2017.

> Researchers report that easily obtainable, over-the-counter mouthwash (Listerine) may prove to be an effective treatment for some cases of gonorrhea.

Clement, Meredith E., and Charles B. Hicks. 2016. "Syphilis on the Rise: What Went Wrong?" *JAMA*, 315(21): 2281-2283. Full text available online at http://www.commed.vcu.edu/IntroPH/Communicable_Disease/2016/JAMA_STI_June.pdf. Accessed on February 8, 2017.

> The authors take note that, as recently as 2000, "eradication of *Treponema pallidum* infection in the United States seemed quite possible." Since that time, however, the rate of infections in the United States has increased significantly. They examine possible reasons for that change.

Clement, Meredith E., N. Lance Okeke, and Charles B. Hicks. 2014. "Treatment of Syphilis: A Systematic Review." *JAMA*, 312(18): 1905-1917. Full text available at http://svmi.web.ve/wh/intertips/SIFILIS-2015.pdf. Accessed on February 8, 2017.

> The authors review 102 articles on the treatment of syphilis published between 1965 and 2014. They examine in particular treatment of specialized populations, such as those individuals infected with HIV. They find that "the mainstay of syphilis treatment is parenteral penicillin G despite the relatively modest clinical trial data that support its use."

Craig, Andrew P., et al. "The Potential Impact of Vaccination on the Prevalence of Gonorrhea." *Vaccine*, 33(36): 4520-4525.

> The authors model the potential effects of a new gonorrhea vaccine in terms of its individual efficacy and its tendency to affect the incidence of gonorrhea in the general

population. They conclude that "a vaccine of moderate efficacy and duration could have a substantive impact on gonococcal prevalence, and disease sequelae, if coverage is high and protection lasts over the highest risk period (i.e., most sexual partner change) among young people."

De Brum, Patricia, Vieira, Tiana Tasca, and W. Evan Secor. 2017. "Challenges and Persistent Questions in the Treatment of Trichomoniasis." *Current Topics in Medicinal Chemistry*, 17(11): 1249-1265.
    This article provides a very good introduction to the issue of trichomoniasis infections and the current state of prevention and treatment for the disease.

Decker, Catherine F., et al. 2016. "Sexually Transmitted Diseases." *Disease-a-Month*, 62(8): 257–318. Available online at http://www.diseaseamonth.com/issue/S0011-5029(15)X0021-6. Accessed on April 3, 2017.
    The August 2016 issue of this journal is devoted completely to a review of the current status of all STIs of any current interest. Each of the nine articles is written by Decker and a collaborator and they provide excellent general introductions to the infections.

De Vries, Henry John C. 2016. "The Enigma of Lymphogranuloma Venereum Spread in Men Who Have Sex with Men." *Sexually Transmitted Diseases*, 43(7): 420-422.
    The author raises the question as to how a disease that has historically been restricted to tropical zones has recently begun to appear in Western Europe, and almost exclusively among men who have sex with men.

Dixon, Alan F. 2015. "Human Sexual Behavior and the Origins of Gonorrhea." *Archives of Sexual Behaviour*, 44(7): 1741-1742.
    The author explores the hypothesis that gonorrhea may have originated in the human species along with the first experiences with oral sex.

Echeverría, Virginia Iommi. 2010. "Girolamo Fracastoro and the Invention of Syphilis." *SciELO.* http://www.scielo.br/pdf/hcsm/v17n4/en_02.pdf. Accessed on March 31, 2017.

This excellent article reviews the life and work of Girolamo Fracastoro, along with an analysis of his contribution to the study of syphilis.

Gannon-Loew, Kathryn, Cynthia Holland-Howe, and Andrea A. Bonny. 2017. "A Review of Expedited Partner Therapy for the Management of Sexually Transmitted Infections in Adolescents." *Journal of Pediatric and Adolescent Gynecology.* http://dx.doi.org/10.1016/j.jpag.2017.01.012. Available online at http://www.sciencedirect.com/science/article/pii/S1083318816302765. Accessed on March 29, 2017.

This article provides a review of "the current literature regarding EPT effectiveness, patients' attitudes and acceptance of EPT, and providers' views and practices surrounding the use of this method of partner treatment."

Gottlieb, Sami L., and Christine Johnson. 2017. "Future Prospects for New Vaccines against Sexually Transmitted Infections." *Current Opinion in Infectious Diseases,* 30(1): 77-86. Available online at http://journals.lww.com/co-infectiousdiseases/Fulltext/2017/02000/Future_prospects_for_new_vaccines_against_sexually.11.aspx. Accessed on March 29, 2017.

This article provides a good general review of the development of vaccines for STIs to the present time, with prospects for vaccines against other infections such as the herpes simplex 1 virus (HSV-1), *Chlamydia trachomatis*, *Neisseria gonorrhoeae*, and *Treponema pallidum*.

Guidry, J. T., and R. S. Scott. 2017. "The Interaction between Human Papillomavirus and Other Viruses." *Virus Research,* 231: 139-147.

The authors point out that human papillomavirus (HPV) is a necessary, but not sufficient, causative agent for the forms of cancer with which it is often associated. They discuss how the presence of other agents, such as HIV, HSV-1, HSV-2, human cytomegalovirus, Epstein–Barr virus, and adeno-associated virus, also plays a role in the carcinogenic action of HPV.

Harper, Kristin N., et al. 2011. "The Origin and Antiquity of Syphilis Revisited: An Appraisal of Old World Pre-Columbian Evidence for Treponemal Infection." *American Journal of Physical Anthropology*, 146(S53): 99-133.

The authors conducted a comprehensive survey of the literature in an effort to provide conclusive evidence for the New World versus Old World controversy about the origin of syphilis. They report that they "did not find a single case of Old World treponemal disease that has both a certain diagnosis and a secure pre-Columbian date."

Holman, Dawn M., et al. 2014. "Barriers to Human Papillomavirus Vaccination among US Adolescents: A Systematic Review of the Literature." *JAMA Pediatrics*, 168(1): 76-82. Available online at https://www.ncbi.nlm.nih.gov/pmc/articles/PMC4538997/. Accessed on March 29, 2017.

The authors find that greater use of the HPV vaccine can be attributed to a number of factors, including lack of adequate information among parents, concerns about the vaccine's effect on sexual behavior, low perceived risk of HPV infection, social influences, irregular preventive care, and vaccine cost.

Ingram, Brooke. 2016. "The Many Presentations of Syphilis." *Journal of the Dermatology Nurses' Association*, 8(5): 318-324.

Ingram briefly reviews the nature of the disease and then focuses on the variety of ways in which the disease can present at various stages (primary, secondary, and tertiary) of the disease.

Jerse, Ann E., Margaret C. Bash, and Michael W. 2014. "Vaccines against Gonorrhea: Current Status and Future Challenges." *Vaccine*, 32(14): 1579-1587.

The authors discuss the need for a gonorrhea vaccine, the problems related to the development of such a vaccine, and the current status of vaccine research.

Kidd, Sarah, and Kimberly A. Workowski. 2015. "Management of Gonorrhea in Adolescents and Adults in the United States." *Clinical Infectious Diseases*, 61(Suppl 8): S785-S780.

This article summarizes discussions about and recommendations for the treatment of gonorrhea in adolescents and adults in the United States. It is based on the Sexually Transmitted Diseases (STD) Treatment Guidelines Expert Consultation meeting in April 2013, which considered nine specific questions about the treatment process.

Korzeniewski, Krzysztof, and Dariusz Juszczak. 2015. "Travel-Related Sexually Transmitted Infections." *International Maritime Health*, 66(4): 238-246. Available online at https://journals.viamedica.pl/international_maritime_health/article/view/IMH.2015.0045/30575. Accessed on April 3, 2017.

The authors discuss the special risks posed by individuals who travel to foreign countries and engage in casual sexual encounters in those countries. They focus on the epidemiology and characteristics signs and symptoms of all major STIs.

Leruez-Ville, Marianne, and Yves Ville. 2017. "Fetal Cytomegalovirus Infection." *Best Practice & Research Clinical Obstetrics & Gynaecology*, 38: 97–107.

While the rate of cytomegalovirus infection among newborn children is about 0.7 percent worldwide, no reliable and consistent protocols have as yet been established for the testing of women at risk for the disease prior to birth of their children. The article discusses this problem.

Levine, G. 1991. "Sexually Transmitted Parasitic Diseases." *Primary Care*, 18(1): 101-128.
> This somewhat dated article is still among the very best expositions on the nature of non-STI diseases that can be transmitted by sexual contact. They include amebiasis, gardiasis, trichomoniasis, scabies, and pubic lice.

Lewis, David A. 2014. "Epidemiology, Clinical Features, Diagnosis and Treatment of Haemophilus Ducreyi—A Disappearing Pathogen?" *Expert Review of Anti-infective Therapy*, 12(6): 687-696.
> The author takes note of the fact that chancroid may be disappearing as a serious disease threat in most parts of the world, including regions where it was previously endemic. He then reviews current options for treatment of the disease and notes that little or no research on new treatments is being conducted.

Ligon, B. Lee. 2005. "Albert Ludwig Sigesmund Neisser: Discoverer of the Cause of Gonorrhea." *Seminars in Pediatric Infectious Diseases*, 16(4): 336–341.
> This article provides a brief, but interesting, biography of the discoverer of the causative agent for gonorrhea.

Lindeman, Zachary, et al. 2014. "Assessing the Antibiotic Potential of Essential Oils against *Haemophilus ducreyi. BMC Complementary and Alternative Medicine*, 14(1): art172, 1-4. Available online at http://bmccomplementalternmed.biomedcentral.com/articles/10.1186/1472-6882-14-172. Accessed on April 2, 2017.
> The authors report that three essential oils, *Cinnamomum verum* (cinnamon), *Eugenia caryophyllus* (clove), and *Thymus satureioides* (thyme) are effective against nine strains of *Haemophilus ducreyi*, and found them all to be significantly effective in killing the bacterium.

Lithgow, Karen V., and Caroline E. Cameron. 2017. "Vaccine Development for Syphilis." *Expert Review of Vaccines*, 16(1): 37-44.

The authors review the need for a vaccine for syphilis, previous efforts to develop such a vaccine, and the current status of research on a vaccine.

Majewska, Anna, et al. 2015. "Antiviral Medication in Sexually Transmitted Diseases. Part II: HIV." *Mini-Reviews in Medicinal Chemistry*, 15(2): 93-103.

Majewska, Anna, et al. 2017. "Antiviral Medication in Sexually Transmitted Diseases. Part III: Hepatitis B, Hepatitis C." *Mini-Reviews in Medicinal Chemistry*, 17(4): 328-337.
The above two articles by Anna Majewska provide a detailed, comprehensive, and technical review of the special challenges presented by STDs causes by viral agents and progress in developing methods of treatments for such infections.

Marks, Michael. 2016. "Yaws: Towards the WHO Eradication Target." *Transactions of the Royal Society of Tropical Medicine and Hygiene*, 110(6): 319-320. Available online at https://academic.oup.com/trstmh/article/110/6/319/1753228/Yaws-towards-the-WHO-eradication-target. Accessed on April 3, 2017.
This article provides a useful general overview of a non-STI relative of syphilis, yaws. It describes current WHO efforts to eradicate the disease worldwide by the year 2020.

Marks, Michael, et al. 2015. "Yaws." *International Journal of STD and AIDS*, 26(10): 696-703.
The authors provide a good, general introduction to a disease caused by a strain of the Treponema bacterium, *T. pallidum* subspecies *pertenue*.

Martin, Natasha K., et al. 2013. "Combination Interventions to Prevent HCV Transmission among People Who Inject Drugs: Modeling the Impact of Antiviral Treatment, Needle and Syringe

Programs, and Opiate Substitution Therapy." *Clinical Infectious Diseases*, 57(suppl2): S39-S45.

The authors review existing evidence on methods for reducing the transmission of hepatitis C virus among people who inject drugs. They conclude that the most effective program involves a needle exchange program, opiate substitution therapy, and treatment with antiviral medications.

Mehriardestani, Mozhgan, et al. 2017. "Medicinal Plants and Their Isolated Compounds Showing Anti-Trichomonas vaginalis-Activity." *Biomedicine & Pharmacotherapy*, 88(3): 885-893.

The authors take note of the fact that *Trichomonas vaginalis* is a major causative agent for a variety of common STDs and that the organism is developing resistance to the only chemical options for treatment, the nitroimidazoles. They suggest that it may be possible to find botanical substitutes for this family of compounds and survey the literature for information on such options. They find three plants, *Persea americana*, *Ocimum basilicum*, and *Verbascum thapsus*, with proven therapeutic value and suggest further research aimed at expanding the number of botanical options that may be effective against *T. vaginalis*.

Mlynarczyk-Bonikowska, Beata, et al. 2013. "Antiviral Medication in Sexually Transmitted Diseases. Part I: HSV, HPV." *Mini-Reviews in Medicinal Chemistry*, 13(13): 1837-1845.

This article provides a detailed, comprehensive, and technical review of the special challenges presented by STDs causes by viral agents and progress in developing methods of treatments for such infections.

Mogha, Kanchan V., and Jashbhai B. Prajapati. 2016. Probiotics for Treating Bacterial Vaginosis." *Reviews in Medical Microbiology*, 27(3): 87–94.

The authors test the efficacy of using probiotics in a variety of ways to reduce a woman's risk for developing bacterial vaginosis.

Morton, R. S. 1968. "Another Look at the *Morbus Gallicus*." *British Journal of Venereal Disease*, 44(174): 174–177.
This article brings together much of the early evidence that points to the original of syphilis in the New World, not in Europe, as some authorities had look contended.

Nasioudis, D., et al. 2017. "Bacterial Vaginosis: A Critical Analysis of Current Knowledge." *BJOG*, 124(1): 61-69.
This article provides a comprehensive review of all that is known about bacterial vaginosis as of 2017.

O'Byrne, Patrick, et al. 2016. "Clinical Review: Approach to Lymphogranuloma Venereum." *Canadian Family Physician*, 62(7): 554-558.
The authors take note that a disease that was once almost entirely one of tropical areas has now begun to spread through western Europe, the United States, Australia, and Canada. They review the characteristic features of the disease and the treatments available for it.

Onderdonk, Andrew B., Mary L. Delaney, and Raina N. Fichorova. 2016. "The Human Microbiome during Bacterial Vaginosis." *Clinical Microbiology Reviews*, 29(2): 223-238. Available online at http://cmr.asm.org/content/29/2/223.long. Accessed on April 2, 2017.
This article provides an excellent general introduction to and overview of bacterial vaginosis infections, along with an extended discussion of the nature of the microbiomes in pregnant and nonpregnant women.

Otto, Robert B., Sarah Ameso, and Bernadina Onegi. 2014. "Assessment of Antibacterial Activity of Crude Leaf and Root

Extracts of Cassia alata against Neisseria gonorrhea." *African Health Sciences*, 14(4): 840–848. Available online at https://www.ncbi.nlm.nih.gov/pmc/articles/PMC4370063/. Accessed on April 1, 2017.

This paper reports on a study attempting to determine the effectiveness of a natural product (the *Cassia Alata* plant) on the *Neisseria gonorrhea* bacterium. The authors conclude that "both the leaf and the root of Cassia alata plant have activity against clinically resistant Neisseria gonorrhoeae."

Pearson, William S., et al. 2017. "Increase in Urgent Care Center Visits for Sexually Transmitted Infections, United States, 2010–2014." *Emerging Infectious Diseases*, 23(2): 367-369.

This article provides a brief statistical overview of the trends in visits related to STIs to urgent care facilities in the United States.

Peterman, Thomas A., et al. 2016. "Gonorrhea Control, United States, 1972–2015: A Narrative Review." *Sexually Transmitted Diseases*, 43(12): 725-730.

This article summarizes trends in the incidence of gonorrhea in the United States over four decades, noting changing attitudes and practices toward control of the disease and reasons for these changes.

Rac, Martha W. F., Paula A. Revell, and Catherine S. Eppes. 2017. "Syphilis during Pregnancy: A Preventable Threat to Maternal–Fetal Health." *American Journal of Obstetrics and Gynecology*, 216(4): 352-363.

The authors remind readers of the problems associated with prospective mothers who are infected with syphilis. They recommend a number of steps that should be taken among pregnant women before delivery occurs.

Schneider, Karl, et al. 2016. "Screening for Asymptomatic Gonorrhea and Chlamydia in the Pediatric Emergency Department." *Sexually*

Transmitted Diseases, 43(4): 209–215. Available online at http://journals.lww.com/stdjournal/Fulltext/2016/04000/Screening_for_Asymptomatic_Gonorrhea_and_Chlamydia.1.aspx. Accessed on March 31, 2017.

    Researchers studied 403 adolescents who visited a pediatric emergency department for non-STI-related health problems to determine the presence of asymptomatic gonorrhea and chlamydia. They found that just under 10 percent of those individuals tested positive for one or the other (or both) infection. The rate among non-white subjects was about six times as great as that for white volunteers.

Schwebke, Jane R., et al. 2016. "Home Screening for Bacterial Vaginosis to Prevent Sexually Transmitted Diseases." *Clinical Infectious Diseases*, 62(5): 531-536. Available online at https://academic.oup.com/cid/article/62/5/531/2462939/Home-Screening-for-Bacterial-Vaginosis-to-Prevent. Accessed on April 2, 2017.

    This paper reports on a study of 1,365 women who agreed to use a home testing kit to determine their bacterial vaginosis status and their development of STIs. The home test seems to be an effective way of detecting asymptomatic bacterial vaginosis.

Shelton, Andrew A. 2004. "Sexually Transmitted Diseases of the Colon, Rectum, and Anus." *Clinics in Colon and Rectal Surgery*, 17(4): 231–234. Available online at https://www.ncbi.nlm.nih.gov/pmc/articles/PMC2780057/#__sec1title. Accessed on April 4, 2017.

    This older article provides valuable information that is still helpful on two less frequently discussed STIs, amebiasis and giardiasis.

Shiadeh, Malihe Nourollahpour, et al. 2016. "Human Parasitic Protozoan Infection to Infertility: A Systematic Review." *Parasitology Research*, 115(2): 469-477.

This article focuses on a variety of intestinal parasites, some of which are transmitted by sexual conduct, and their effects on fertility.

Skapinyecz, J., et al. 2003. "Pelvic Inflammatory Disease Is a Risk Factor for Cervical Cancer." *European Journal of Gynaecological Oncology*, 24(5): 401-404.

This paper is of historical interest because it is one of the earliest (if not the earliest) report providing conclusive evidence of the connection between pelvic inflammatory disease (PID) and cervical cancer.

Stamm, Lola V., and Angel A. Noda. 2017. "Elimination of Mother-to-Child Transmission of Syphilis in the Americas—A Goal That Must Not Slip Away." *Sexually Transmitted Diseases*, 44(1): 12-13.

This editorial commentary takes note of worldwide efforts to end the threat of congenital syphilis, reviews the reasons behind this international campaign, and explains the steps that need to be taken to achieve this objective.

Talukdar, Joy. 2012. "The History of Sexually Transmitted Diseases." *International Journal of Medical and Health Sciences*, 1(3): 83–88. Also available online at http://www.ijmhs.net/articles/1342356709The_History_of_Sexually_Transmitted_Diseases.pdf. Accessed on February 2, 2017.

Talukdar discusses the history of STIs from the medieval period to the present day, with some attention to the rise of modern "second" and "third" generation STIs, such as hepatitis and HIV/AIDS.

Taylor-Robinson, David, and Jørgen Skov Jensen. 2011. "*Mycoplasma genitalium*: From Chrysalis to Multicolored Butterfly." *Clinical Microbiology Reviews*, 24(3): 498–514. Available online at https://www.ncbi.nlm.nih.gov/pmc/articles/PMC3131060/. Accessed on April 3, 2017.

This comprehensive essay on *Mycoplasma genitalium* includes a review of its discovery and early history, biological and physical characteristics, genetic structure, pathogenesis, detection, and related diseases in men and women.

Tetteh, Raymond A., et al. 2017. "Pre-Exposure Prophylaxis for HIV Prevention: Safety Concerns." *Drug Safety*, 40(4): 273–283.
The authors conduct a meta-analysis of studies dealing with the safety of the PrEP medication tenofovir disoproxil fumarate/emtricitabine (Truvada®) and find that no serious adverse effects have been associated with use of the drug. They also discover that the minor adverse effects are generally associated with gastrointestinal issues, such as mild to moderate nausea, vomiting, and diarrhea.

Tsevat, Danielle G., et al. 2017. "Sexually Transmitted Diseases and Infertility." *American Journal of Obstetrics and Gynecology*, 216(1): 1-9. Available online at http://www.ajog.org/article/S0002-9378(16)30573-7/pdf. Accessed on February 8, 2017.
The authors note that most cases of tubal factor infertility worldwide are caused by undiagnosed STDs. They review the mechanisms by which such infections occur, the possible involvement of other causative agents, and the need for further research aimed at reducing this serious public health problem.

Unemo, Magnus, and Jorgen S. Jensen. 2017. "Antimicrobial-Resistant Sexually Transmitted Infections: Gonorrhoea and *Mycoplasma genitalium*." *Nature Reviews. Urology*, 14(3): 139-152. Available online at http://www.nature.com/nrurol/journal/v14/n3/full/nrurol.2016.268.html. Accessed on March 29, 2017.
The authors discuss the appearance and spread of drug-resistant forms of *N. gonorrhoeae* and *M. genitalium*, the reasons for this problem, ultimate consequences of its not

being brought under control, and mechanisms by which the problem might be resolved.

Wangu, Zoon, and Gale R. Burstein. 2017. "Adolescent Sexuality: Updates to the Sexually Transmitted Infection Guidelines." *Pediatric Clinics of North America*, 64(2): 389-411.

This article reviews the STIs to which adolescents may be exposed and discusses the latest revision in Centers for Disease Control and Prevention (CDC) guidelines for the prevention, screening, diagnosis, and management of STIs in this population.

White, Mark Donald. 2014. "Pros, Cons, and Ethics of HPV Vaccine in Teens—Why Such Controversy?" *Translational Andrology and Urology*, 3(4): 429-434.

The author reports on a survey of online articles about the use of and attitudes toward the HPV vaccine and summarizes the reasons he thinks the topic is surrounded by such debate and controversy.

Woolston, Sophie L., Shireesha Dhanireddy, and Jeanne Marrazzo. 2016. "Ocular Syphilis: A Clinical Review." *Current Infectious Disease Reports*, 18(11): 1-6.

This article provides a general overview of syphilitic infections of the eye.

Reports

Cantor, Amy G., et al. 2016. "Screening for Syphilis: Updated Evidence Report and Systematic Review for the US Preventive Services Task Force." U.S. Preventive Services Task Force. *JAMA*, 315(21): 2328-2337.

This report is an update of a 2004 review of the effectiveness of syphilis screening programs, test accuracy, and harms to nonpregnant adults and adolescents of such programs. The study concludes that "screening algorithms with high sensitivity and specificity are available to accurately detect syphilis," "treatment with antibiotics can lead to substantial health benefits in nonpregnant persons who are at increased risk for syphilis infection by curing syphilis infection, preventing manifestations of late-stage disease, and preventing sexual transmission to others," and "no direct evidence on the harms of screening for syphilis in nonpregnant persons who are at increased risk for infection."

Centers for Disease Control and Prevention. 2016. *Sexually Transmitted Disease Surveillance 2015*. Atlanta: U.S. Department of Health and Human Services. Available online at https://www.cdc.gov/std/stats15/std-surveillance-2015-print.pdf. Accessed on March 29, 2017.

This report provides what is probably the most extensive and complete statistical information about the status of STI diseases in the United States, including some important historical data.

Cunningham, Scott, and Manisha Shah. 2014. "Decriminalizing Indoor Prostitution: Implications for Sexual Violence and Public Health." NBER Working Paper No. 20281. National Bureau of Economic Research. http://www.nber.org/papers/w20281. Accessed on April 1, 2017.

This working paper discusses the effects on public health and sexual crime issues of an inadvertent court ruling in Rhode Island in 2003 that essentially legalized prostitution. The authors report that, following that ruling, rape decreased by 31 percent and female gonorrhea rates by 39 percent in the general population in the state.

"Final Recommendation Statement: Chlamydia and Gonorrhea: Screening." 2014. U.S. Preventive Services Task Force. https://

www.uspreventiveservicestaskforce.org/Page/Document/
RecommendationStatementFinal/chlamydia-and-gonorrhea-
screening. Accessed on April 1, 2017.

This document summarizes the U.S. Preventive Services
Task Force's (USPSTF) recommendations for screening programs for gonorrhea and chlamydia, including
populations served, clinical considerations, and other
considerations.

"Final Report of the National Medical Association, Tuskegee
Syphilis Study Ad Hoc Committee." National Medical Association.
Tuskegee Syphilis Study Ad Hoc Committee. http://www.
research.usf.edu/dric/hrpp/foundations-course/docs/finalreport-
tuskegeestudyadvisorypanel.pdf. Accessed on April 5, 2017.

A committee was appointed to investigate the details of
the now-infamous Tuskegee syphilis study that ran from
1932 to 1972. The committee was authorized by Section 222 of the Public Health Service Act, as amended, 42
US Code 217a, and provisions of Executive Order 11671.
The specific charge of the committee was to (1) determine
whether the study was justified in 1932 and whether it
should have been continued when penicillin became generally available; (2) recommend whether the study should
be continued at this point in time, and if not, how it
should be terminated in a way consistent with the rights
and health needs of its remaining participants; and (3)
determine whether existing policies to protect the rights
of patients participating in health research conducted or
supported by the Department of Health, Education, and
Welfare are adequate and effective and to recommend
improvements in these policies, if needed.

"New Jersey Syringe Access Program Demonstration Project.
Final Report." 2012. Trenton, NJ: New Jersey Department of
Health. Available online at https://dspace.njstatelib.org/xmlui/

bitstream/handle/10929/29746/h4342012a.pdf?sequence=1. Accessed on April 5, 2017.

The New Jersey state legislature passed the Bloodborne Disease Harm Reduction Act of 2006 (P.L. 2006, c. 99), providing for the creation and operation of up to six needle exchange programs in the state. This report summarizes information gained about needle exchange programs in the prevention of STDs for the five centers that were actually created. The report recommended that the program be continued and expanded in some ways, where finances permitted.

Shafer, J. K., Lida J. Usilton, and Geraldine A. Gleeson. 1954. "Untreated Syphilis in the Male Negro—A Prospective Study of the Effect on Life Expectancy." *Public Health Reports*, 69(7): 684–690. Available online at https://www.ncbi.nlm.nih.gov/pmc/articles/PMC2024307/pdf/pubhealthreporig00175-0078.pdf. Accessed on April 5, 2017.

For readers interested in technical details of the Tuskegee syphilis study, this report provides a paper typical of the reports arising out of the research.

Zahker, Bernadette, et al. 2014. "Screening for Gonorrhea and Chlamydia: A Systematic Review for the U.S. Preventive Services Task Force." *Annals of Internal Medicine*, 161(12): 884-893. Available online at http://annals.org/aim/article/1906845/screening-gonorrhea-chlamydia-systematic-review-u-s-preventive-services-task. Accessed on March 31, 2017.

This review is the most recent report for the USPSTF on the effectiveness and risk factors related to screening programs for gonorrhea and chlamydia in populations previously recommended for such testing by the USPSTF. Among the study conclusions was the observation that "screening for chlamydia may reduce the incidence of PID in young women."

Internet

Aicken, Catherine R. H., et al. 2016. "Young People's Perceptions of Smartphone-Enabled Self-Testing and Online Care for Sexually Transmitted Infections: Qualitative Interview Study." *BMC Public Health*. http://bmcpublichealth.biomedcentral.com/ articles/10.1186/s12889-016-3648-y. Accessed on March 30, 2017.

Adolescents report a number of factors that contribute to their hesitancy to seek professional help for possible sexually transmitted infections, including "embarrassment regarding face-to-face consultations; the time-commitment needed to attend clinic; privacy concerns (e.g. being seen attending clinic); and issues related to confidentiality." A program has been developed through which young adults can obtain this information through use of their cell phones. This article examines adolescent attitudes toward the new system.

Alexander, Krystal. 2016. "Working toward a Vaccine for Chlamydia." American Council on Science and Health. http:// acsh.org/news/2016/07/21/working-toward-a-vaccine-for-chlamydia. Accessed on April 1, 2017.

This web page provides a simplified report on the development of a vaccine for chlamydia at Bulir et al., 2016, *q.v.* above.

"Amebiasis." 2017. *MedlinePlus*. https://medlineplus.gov/ency/ article/000298.htm. Accessed on April 4, 2017.

This web page is one of the best general introductions to a STI caused by the parasite *Entamoeba histolytica*.

Andrews, Michelle. 2017. "New Vaccine Recommendation Cuts Number of HPV Shots Children Need." *Kaiser Health News*. http:// khn.org/news/new-vaccine-recommendation-cuts-number-of-hpv-shots-children-need/. Accessed on March 29, 2017.

This article reports on changes recently made by the CDC with regard to the number and timing of HPV shots recommended for boys and girls. It also discusses some of the issues involved with making the inoculation more popular among the general public.

Blondeel, Karel, et al. 2016. "Evidence and Knowledge Gaps on the Disease Burden in Sexual and Gender Minorities: A Review of Systematic Reviews." *International Journal for Equity in Health*. https://equityhealthj.biomedcentral.com/articles/10.1186/s12939-016-0304--. Accessed on March 30, 2017.

This article explores the generally held notion that individuals with a variety of nontypical sexual orientations, gender identities and expressions, and physical characteristics tend to have a higher rate of STIs than do the general population. The authors examine a number of meta-analyses on this issue and conclude that the belief is largely confirmed in research studies, along with a lower level of knowledge and understanding among such groups as to the characteristics of STIs.

Bloom, Josh. 2016. "How Do Herpes Drugs Work?" American Council on Science and Health. http://acsh.org/news/2016/08/30/how-do-herpes-drugs-work-9941. Accessed on April 5, 2017.

This moderately technical article provides a clear and understandable explanation as to the biochemical changes that occur when some type of drug is used against the herpes virus.

Borgobello, Bridget. 2014. "Innovative Soho Clinic Streamlines Sexual Health Testing." *New Atlas*. http://newatlas.com/nhs-dean-street-express-clinic-london-penson/32071/. Accessed on March 29, 2017.

This web page describes an innovative way for London residents to obtain fast, accurate, private STI tests by visiting health units within the city capable of helping individuals conduct such tests on their own.

Branswell, Helen. 2016. "Gonorrhea May Soon Become Resistant to All Antibiotics and Untreatable." *Stat*. https://www.statnews. com/2016/07/14/gonorrhea-antibiotic-resistant-untreatable/. Accessed on March 31, 2017.

    The author reviews recent history of gonorrhea treatment and notes that the disease is becoming resistant to antibiotics that have traditionally been used for its cure.

"Centers for Disease Control and Prevention (CDC) Program Guidance for Implementing Certain Components of Syringe Services Programs, 2016." 2016. Centers for Disease Control and Prevention. https://www.cdc.gov/hiv/pdf/risk/cdc-hiv-syringe-exchange-services.pdf. Accessed on April 5, 2017.

    This publication outlines the role that the federal government (through the CDC) can play in the creation and development of needle exchange programs.

Chavoustie, S. E., et al. 2017. "Experts Explore the State of Bacterial Vaginosis and the Unmet Needs Facing Women and Providers." *International Journal of Gynaecology and Obstetrics*. http://onlinelibrary.wiley.com/doi/10.1002/ijgo.12114/full. Accessed on April 1, 2017.

    This article is a report on a 2016 meeting of "nine women's health leaders" from across the United States. The meeting resulted in a consensus statement about the status and treatment of bacterial vaginosis and key findings developed by the group.

Cock, Emily. 2017. "'He Would by No Means Risque His Reputation': Patient and Doctor Shame in Daniel Turner's De Morbis Cutaneis (1714) and Syphilis (1717)." *Medical Humanities*. http://mh.bmj.com/content/early/2017/01/17/medhum-

2016-011057. Accessed on March 31, 2017. (Epub ahead of publication.)

> Embarrassment and shame have always been associated with STIs. This article describes one of the earliest observations on the ways in which these emotional responses affected the work of one of the best known of early researchers.

Crain, Esther. "What's the Difference between STDs and STIs?" *Women's Health.* http://www.womenshealthmag.com/health/sti-vs-std. Accessed on April 5, 2017.

> The author explains the very real difference between the two terms *sexually transmitted diseases* and *sexually transmitted infections.*

"Cryptosporidium Enteritis." 2017. *MedlinePlus.* https://medlineplus.gov/ency/article/000617.htm. Accessed on April 4, 2017.

> Although commonly spread by mechanisms other than sexual activities, cryptosporidium enteritis can also be transmitted during sex between two men and especially when one or both members of a sexual activity are immune-suppressed, as with those who are HIV positive.

"Debate: Needle Exchanges." 2011. *Debatepedia.* http://debatepedia.idebate.org/en/index.php/Debate:_Needle_exchanges. Accessed on April 5, 2017.

> This website brings together a number of arguments both for and against the use of needle exchange programs. The arguments are generally presented in considerable detail with every possible angle in the debate described.

"Directory of Syringe Exchange Programs." 2017. NASEN. North American Syringe Exchange Network. https://nasen.org/directory/. Accessed on April 5, 2017.

This web page, provided by NASEN, allows an individual to find the location of a needle exchange program in any one of the 50 states, the District of Columbia, or Puerto Rico.

"Effective HIV and STD Prevention Programs for Youth: A Summary of Scientific Evidence." 2010. Centers for Disease Control and Prevention. https://www.cdc.gov/healthyyouth/ sexualbehaviors/pdf/effective_hiv.pdf. Accessed on April 5, 2017.

This pamphlet summarizes the best information currently available with regard to the principles on which an STI prevention program should be based.

"Expedited Partner Therapy." 2017. Centers for Disease Control and Prevention. https://www.cdc.gov/std/ept/. Accessed on April 5, 2017.

This web page provides good introductory information and many useful resources about the topic of expedited partner therapy, including guidance on the development of such programs, legal issues that may be involved, research findings, and insurance billing for such programs.

Field, Scott S. 2016. "New Concerns about Human Papillomavirus Vaccine." American College of Pediatrics. https://www.acpeds. org/wordpress/wp-content/uploads/1.26.16-New-Concerns- about-the-HPV-vaccine.pdf. Accessed on February 9, 2017.

This press release summarizes recent research on the safety of the HPV vaccine, and discusses four specific issues regarding use of the vaccine that still require additional research. The purpose of the press release is to make individuals considering the use of the vaccine "aware of these concerns pending further action by the regulatory agencies and manufacturers."

"First Evidence Drug Used to Combat Malaria in Pregnancy Also Protects against Sexually Transmitted Infections." 2017.

London School of Hygiene and Tropical Medicine. http://www.lshtm.ac.uk/newsevents/news/2017/drug_malaria_pregnancy_protects_against_sti.html. Accessed on March 29, 2017.

> The report describes recent clinical findings that a drug used to prevent malaria among pregnant women also appears to reduce their risk for contracting STIs.

Flannery, Maura. 2017. "Historic Dispute: Did Syphilis Originate in the New World, from Which It Was Brought to Europe by Christopher Columbus and His Crew?" *Science Clarified*. http://www.scienceclarified.com/dispute/Vol-2/Historic-Dispute-Did-syphilis-originate-in-the-New-World-from-which-it-was-brought-to-Europe-by-Christopher-Columbus-and-his-crew.html#ixzz4RnTSaihp. Accessed on February 9, 2017.

> This article provides a nice general introduction to the dispute over the possible origins of syphilis in Europe and throughout the rest of the world.

"Giardia Infection." 2017. *MedlinePlus*. https://medlineplus.gov/ency/article/000288.htm. Accessed on April 4, 2017.

> Strictly speaking, giardia infections are not STIs because they are most commonly transmitted by means other than sexual activities between two individuals, although sexual activity is one mechanism by which they can be transmitted. This web page provides an excellent overview of the disease that is mentioned less often than syphilis, gonorrhea, chlamydia, and some other STIs.

Gompf, Sandra Gonzalez. 2016. "Cytomegalovirus (CMV) Infection." MedicineNet.com. http://www.medicinenet.com/cytomegalovirus_cmv/article.htm. Accessed on April 3, 2017.

> This essay discusses cytomegalovirus infections in detail, providing information on the biological nature of the organism, methods of transmission, diagnosis, and treatment of the disease.

Gonzalez-Astudillo, Viviana, et al. 2017. Decline Causes of Koalas in South East Queensland, Australia: A 17-year Retrospective Study of Mortality and Morbidity." *Scientific Reports*. 7. Article number: 42587. doi:10.1038/srep42587.

> The authors report that the two primary causes of the 80 percent decline in the koala population in Queensland are cars and the spread of chlamydia in the population. The latter factor is a problem because *Chlamydia spp.* infections cause infertility in the females of the species.

Goode, Leslie. 2017. "A New Kind of Treatment for Multi-Resistant Gonorrhoea?" BMJ Blogs. http://blogs.bmj.com/sti/2017/01/31/a-new-kind-of-treatment-for-multi-resistant-gonorrhoea/. Accessed on March 29, 2017.

> This web page provides information on a promising new way of treating gonorrheal infections that makes use of compounds that release carbon monoxide when irradiated. The carbon monoxide appears, even at low levels, to be effective in destroying the *N. gonorrhoeae* microorganism.

Gorman, Anna. 2017. "Spike in Syphilis among Newborns Driven by Broader Epidemic." *Kaiser Health News*. http://khn.org/news/spike-in-syphilis-among-newborns-driven-by-broader-epidemic/. Accessed on March 30, 2017.

> This article deals with an unexpected increase in the number of congenital syphilis cases and its relationship to a general increase in syphilis cases over the past few years.

Grimes, David Robert. 2016. "We Know It's Effective. So Why Is There Opposition to the HPV Vaccine?" *The Guardian*. https://www.theguardian.com/science/blog/2016/jan/11/why-is-there-opposition-hpv-vaccine-cervical-cancer. Accessed on March 29, 2017.

> The author suggests that the answer to this question is at least twofold: (1) people do not like to talk or think about

sexual issues, and (2) incorrect and misleading information about the vaccine's safety has made people fearful of
exposing their children to the vaccine.

Gunter, Jennifer. 2017. "Pubic Hair Grooming Means More
Sexually Transmitted Infections. Why?" KevinMD.com. http://
www.kevinmd.com/blog/2017/01/pubic-hair-grooming-means-
sexually-transmitted-infections.html. Accessed on March 29, 2017.
    Growing numbers of women have adopted the practice of
    pubic hair grooming. The author explains how this practice
    might lead to an increase in the number of STIs that occur.

Haelle, Tara. 2015. "Gardasil HPV Vaccine Safety Assessed in
Most Comprehensive Study to Date." *Forbes.* http://www.forbes.
com/sites/tarahaelle/2015/07/15/gardasil-hpv-vaccine-safety-
assessed-in-most-comprehensive-study-to-date/#4e1fd09c53ad.
Accessed on February 9, 2017.
    This article reports on a large study on the effects and side
    effects of the Gardasil HPV vaccine, results that appear
    to give the vaccine a "clean bill of health." The article is
    of special interest because of other reports that raise ques-
    tions about the safety of the vaccine.

Hahn, Andrew W., and David H. Spach. 2017. "Human
Papilloma Virus." National STD Curriculum. http://www.std.
uw.edu/go/pathogen-based/hpv/core-concept/all. Accessed on
March 29, 2017.
    This website offers what is probably the most complete
    and most detailed discussion of the nature of the HPV, its
    effects on the human body, the use of the HPV vaccine,
    and related issues.

Hirsch, Larissa. 2017. "About Sexually Transmitted Diseases."
Teens Health. https://kidshealth.org/en/teens/std.html#. Accessed
on January 31, 2017.

This website provides information about STIs of special interest to teenagers. It is part of a group of web pages that include information for pre-teens and adults as well.

"An HIV Vaccine: The World's Best Long-Term Hope for Ending AIDS." 2017. HIV Vaccine Trials Network. https://www.hvtn. org/en.html. Accessed on April 5, 2017.

This website provides complete and up-to-date information on the latest advances in research on an HIV vaccine, including the results of recent clinical trials.

"HPV Vaccine." 2017. Planned Parenthood. https://www. plannedparenthood.org/learn/stds-hiv-safer-sex/hpv/hpv-vaccine?_ga=1.88080088.1194818631.1486680060. Accessed on February 9, 2017.

This website provides detailed information on the HPV and the vaccine that is available to prevent HPV infections. It covers topics such as the way in which the vaccine works, how safe the vaccine is, the effects of the vaccine on existing infections, the places the vaccine is available, and its probable cost.

"Human Papilloma Virus." 2016. Centers for Disease Control and Prevention. https://www.cdc.gov/hpv/parents/questions-answers.html. Accessed on March 29, 2017.

This website provides a broad, general introduction to HPV infections and the HPV vaccine, including information about the demographics of the disease, medical problems associated with HPV, methods of HPV transmission, deciding who should get the vaccine, and safety issues associated with the vaccine's use.

Jaxen, Jefferey. 2017. "American College of Pediatricians Latest to Warn of Gardasil HPV Vaccine Dangers." *Vaccine Impact*. https://vaccineimpact.com/2016/american-college-of-pediatricians-latest-to-warn-of-hpv-vaccine-dangers/. Accessed on February 9, 2017.

> The author claims that new evidence is available for growing concerns about the use of the HPV vaccine. He claims that one of the vaccines, Gardasil, has resulted in the sterilization of young women, that scientific research on the vaccine has included fraudulent claims, and that the use of the vaccine has resulted in some deaths among those who have been vaccinated for the infection. The report from the American College of Pediatricians to which he refers in this article can be found at https://www.acpeds. org/wordpress/wp-content/uploads/1.26.16-New-Concerns-about-the-HPV-vaccine.pdf.

Kalichman, Seth C., et al. 2017. "Diminishing Perceived Threat of AIDS and Increasing Sexual Risks of HIV among Men Who Have Sex with Men, 1997–2015." *ResearchGate*. https:// www.researchgate.net/publication/313422029_Diminishing_ Perceived_Threat_of_AIDS_and_Increasing_Sexual_Risks_of_ HIV_Among_Men_Who_Have_Sex_with_Men_1997-2015. Accessed on March 29,2017.

> This article reports on a study as to the ways in which the highly antiretroviral therapy used against HIV infections has negatively affected the views toward sexual activity by men who have sex with men. Such individuals appear to feel safer having unprotected sex now that a reliable treatment is available for the disease.

Kilgrove, Kristina. 2011. "Morbus gallicus in the Roman Empire." Powered by Osteons. http://www.poweredbyosteons. org/2011/10/morbus-gallicus-in-roman-empire.html. Accessed on February 9, 2017.

> This article comments on the (fairly unconvincing) evidence for the existence of syphilis on the European continent prior to 1492, in Rome, in this particular instance.

Knell, Robert J. 2004. "Syphilis in Renaissance Europe: Rapid Evolution of an Introduced Sexually Transmitted Disease?" *Proceedings: The Royal Society. Biology Letters* (Supplement 4): 174-176. https://www.ncbi.nlm.nih.gov/pmc/articles/PMC1810019/pdf/15252975.pdf. Accessed on February 10, 2017.

> This article discusses changes that took place in the syphilis virus in the first few decades following its appearance in Europe, along with social responses to these changes. Within this context, also see Arrizabalaga, Henderson, and French, under Books above.

Leitsch, David. 2017. "Recent Advances in the *Trichomonas vaginalis* Field." *F1000 Research.* https://f1000research.com/articles/5-162/v1. Accessed on April 4, 2017.

> This article discusses recent advances in the epidemiology, pathogenicity, biochemistry, genomics, and treatment of *T. vaginalis* infections.

Lieff, Jon. 2017. "How Do Bacteria Help Cancer?" Searching for the Mind. http://jonlieffmd.com/blog/how-do-bacteria-help-cancer. Accessed on April 1, 2017.

> This article provides a fascinating introduction to the way in which bacteria in the body, including those responsible for certain STIs, produce changes in the body's chemistry and contribute to the risk for a variety of cancers.

Liu, Gui, et al. 2015. "Trends and Patterns of Sexual Behaviors among Adolescents and Adults Aged 14 to 59 Years, United States." *Sexually Transmitted Diseases.* http://journals.lww.com/stdjournal/Fulltext/2015/01000/Trends_and_Patterns_of_Sexual_Behaviors_Among.6.aspx. Accessed on March 30, 2017.

> The authors draw on data collected in the National Health and Nutrition Examination Surveys between 1999 and

2012 to determine trends in the rate of STIs among individuals of different age groups in the United States.

Moi, Harald, Karla Blee, and Patrick J. Horner. 2015. "Management of Non-Gonococcal Urethritis." *BMC Infectious Diseases.* doi:10.1186/s12879-015-1043-4. Available online at https://www.ncbi.nlm.nih.gov/pmc/articles/PMC4518518/. Accessed on March 31, 2017.

This article provides an excellent overview of non-gonococcal urethritis that includes etiology, clinical features and signs, complications, diagnosis, and treatment of the disease.

Murtagh, Maurine M. 2017. "The Point-of-Care Diagnostic Landscape for Sexually Transmitted Infections (STIs)." The Murtagh Group. http://www.who.int/reproductivehealth/topics/rtis/Diagnostic_Landscape_2017.pdf?ua=1. Accessed on March 30, 2017.

This technical article explains what "point-of-care" procedures means for a variety of STIs and the resources that are currently available for conducting such tests.

"National Notifiable Diseases Surveillance System." 2015. Centers for Disease Control and Prevention. https://wwwn.cdc.gov/nndss/. Accessed on April 3, 2017.

This web page explains what the National Notifiable Diseases Surveillance System is and the activities it carries out. It also contains a list of all notifiable diseases, as of 2017.

"New Genital Herpes Vaccine Candidate Provides Powerful Protection in Preclinical Tests." *Science Daily.* https://www.sciencedaily.com/releases/2017/01/170119163444.htm. Accessed on March 30, 2017.

This article reviews the latest information on a possible new vaccine for the treatment of genital herpes.

O'Farrell, Nigel, and Harald Moi. 2016. "2016 European Guideline on Donovanosis." http://www.iusti.org/regions/europe/pdf/2016/Donovanosis2016.pdf. Accessed on April 2, 2017.

These guidelines focus on the diagnosis and management of donovanosis and are published by the International Union against Sexually Transmitted Infections.

Özdener, Ayşe Elif, et al. 2017. "The Future of Pre-Exposure Prophylaxis (PrEP) for Human Immunodeficiency Virus (HIV) Infection." *Expert Review of Anti-infective Therapy.* doi: http://dx.doi.org/10.1080/14787210.2017.1309292. Accessed on April 5, 2017.

The authors discuss the use of a tenofovir disoproxil fumarate/emtricitabine (Truvada®) medication for reducing the risk of HIV infection for individuals who may likely to develop the disease. They also review the status of seven PrEP drugs that are currently in the research and development pipeline for alternatives to the tenofovir disoproxil fumarate/emtricitabine regimen.

Pierce, Jenelle Marie. 2017. "The STD Project's Comprehensive STD List—A List of All STDs." The STD Project. http://www.thestdproject.com/std-list/. Accessed on April 4, 2017.

This excellent website provides basic information on most STIs, including some that are rarely discussed elsewhere, such as *M. genitalium*, scabies, and pubic lice. Links to more detailed information are available, but do NOT selected one of the five labeled bubbles at the beginning of the essay as they take you to nonrelated pages.

"Point-Of-Care Diagnostic Tests (POCTs) for Sexually Transmitted Infections (STIs)." World Health Organization. http://www.who.int/reproductivehealth/topics/rtis/pocts/en/. Accessed on March 30, 2017.

This article explains the process of point-of-care testing for STIs and the current status of the technology for syphilis. (Such tests are not currently available for other STIs.)

"Pubic Lice." 2017. *MedlinePlus*. https://medlineplus.gov/ency/article/000841.htm. Accessed on April 4, 2017.

Pubic lice are tiny insects that are easily transferred during intimate contact between two individuals, one of whom is already infected. Pubic lice cause serious itching, although they are not particularly dangerous to one's health. This website provides basic information on the characteristics of pubic lice, symptoms of an infection, treatment, and prognosis of the disease.

Redelinghuys, Shane, et al. 2015. "Normal Flora and Bacterial Vaginosis in Pregnancy: An Overview." *Critical Reviews in Microbiology*. doi:10.3109/1040841X.2014.954522.

The authors describe the microbiotic status of women during pregnancy, how this can be related to the development of bacterial vaginosis, possible effects on the newborn child, and method for dealing with the condition.

Rettner, Rachel. 2017. "New STD? What You Should Know about Mycoplasma genitalium." *LiveScience*. http://www.livescience.com/52826-mycoplasma-genitalium-std.html. Accessed on March 30, 2017.

This article provides basic information about *M. genitallium* infections, their characteristic features, modes of transmission, and methods of prevention and treatment.

"Scabies." 2017. *MedlinePlus*. https://medlineplus.gov/ency/article/000830.htm. Accessed on April 4, 2017.

Scabies is a highly infectious disease that is easily transmitted from one person to another through the sharing of articles of clothing, bedding, or other materials, or through sexual contact. This web page provides a good general introduction to the causes, symptoms, prognosis, and treatment of the disease.

Scott, Hyman M., and Jeffrey D. Klausner. 2016. "Sexually Transmitted Infections and Pre-Exposure Prophylaxis: Challenges and Opportunities among Men Who Have Sex with Men in the US." *AIDS Research and Therapy*, 13: 5. doi:10.1186/s12981-016-0089-8. https://www.ncbi.nlm.nih.gov/pmc/articles/PMC4719214/. Accessed on March 31, 2017.

> The authors point out that PrEP has been quite successful in reducing the risk of HIV infection among men who have sex with men in the United States. They then note that PrEP may also have success in preventing the transmission of causative agents for other STIs, such as *N. gonorrhoeae*, which have become largely resistant to traditional treatments for the diseases.

Sergio de Carvalho, Newton. 2016. "Sexually Transmitted Infections, Pelvic Inflammatory Disease, and the Role from Intrauterine Devices: Myth or Fact?" *Journal of Biomedical Sciences*. http://www.jbiomeds.com/biomedical-sciences/sexually-transmitted-infections-pelvic-inflammatory-disease-and-the-role-from-intrauterine-devices-myth-or-fact.php?aid=17556. Accessed on March 30, 2017.

> Some researchers have long suspected that the use of intrauterine devices as a means of contraception may increase a woman's risk for pelvic inflammatory disease. This article reviews the empirical evidence on that question and concludes that no such correlation or cause-and-effect relationship appears to exist and that having had an STI is a much greater risk for PID than use of an intrauterine device.

"Sexually Transmitted Diseases." 2017. *Healthy People*. https://www.healthypeople.gov/2020/topics-objectives/topic/sexually-transmitted-diseases. Accessed on January 31, 2017.

Healthy People is a 10-year national campaign designed to improve the overall health of the American people. Among the specific objectives of the program is an effort to "promote healthy sexual behaviors, strengthen community capacity, and increase access to quality services to prevent sexually transmitted diseases (STDs) and their complications." This website provides detailed information about the specific elements of that effort, including the specific types of interventions and resources being used in the effort and "snapshots" of changes in behavior and attitudes that have been measured.

"Sexually Transmitted Diseases." 2017. *MedlinePlus.* https://medlineplus.gov/sexuallytransmitteddiseases.html#cat51. Accessed on January 31, 2017.

This website, a service of the U.S. National Library of Medicine, provides a good overall introduction to the subject of STIs with sections on latest news, symptoms, diagnosis and testing, prevention, treatment, statistics and research, and information for special groups such as men, women, seniors, and teenagers.

"Sexually Transmitted Diseases (STDs)." 2017. Centers for Disease Control and Prevention. https://www.cdc.gov/std/. Accessed on January 31, 2017.

The CDC is one of the primary sources of information about STIs. This web page contains detailed information about the major diseases and related conditions, laboratory information, prevention, management of an STI, projects and initiatives, data and statistics, and treatment for the diseases.

Shaw, Souradet Y. 2016, "Teen Clinics: Missing the Mark? Comparing Pregnancy and Sexually Transmitted Infections Rates among Enrolled and Non-Enrolled Adolescents." *BioMed Central.* https://www.ncbi.nlm.nih.gov/pmc/articles/PMC4915138/. Accessed on March 30, 2017.

The city of Manitoba has established clinics at the city's high school in an effort to reduce rates of both pregnancy and STIs. This study compares the rates of both conditions for (1) students who have access to such clinics, (2) students who do not have access to them, and (3) a similar age cohort consisting of adolescents who are not enrolled in schools. The study found that rates of STIs were much higher for the last of these groups, and higher among those who attend schools *with* clinics compared to those in schools that *do not* have such clinics. The results of the study raise questions about the efficacy of offering STI clinics within a high school.

"STD Awareness: Intestinal Parasites." 2012. Planned Parenthood. http://advocatesaz.org/2012/01/03/sti-awareness-intestinal-parasites/. Accessed on March 30, 2017.

One area of the topic of sexually transmitted infections that is less commonly spoken off involves parasites that are not true STIs, but that can be transmitted during sexual contact. These infections include giardiasis, amebiasis, cryptosporidiosis, pubic lice, and scabies. This article provides an excellent introduction to the characteristics of such diseases.

"STD Prevention Success Stories." 2016. Centers for Disease Control and Prevention. https://www.cdc.gov/std/products/success/default.htm. Accessed on April 5, 2017.

This web page features nine special programs describing successful STD prevention programs in fields such as special campaigns, training of STD workers, antibiotic-resistant gonorrhea, community health approaches, and expedited partner therapy.

Stöppler, Melissa Conrad. 2016. "Sexually Transmitted Diseases (STD)." *emedicinehealth*. http://www.emedicinehealth.com/sexually_transmitted_diseases/article_em.htm. Accessed on February 8, 2017.

This web page provides an excellent general overview of STDs with sections on basic facts; the causes of STDs; and diagnosis, prevention, and treatment for the infections.

"Ten Good Reasons to Be Concerned about the Human Papillomavirus (HPV) Vaccination Campaign." 2008. Women and Health Protection and the Canadian Women's Health Network. http://www.whp-apsf.ca/pdf/Ten%20Good%20Reasons% 20.pdf. Accessed on March 29, 2017.
This summary of reasons for opposing HPV was prepared by La Fédération du Québec pour le Planning Des Naissances (The Quebec Federation for Family Planning) and includes arguments such as there is no epidemic of HPV right now, so no need to have a vaccination, the existing vaccine does not provide full protection against PID, and the vaccine is likely to give women a false sense of security about possible cervical cancer issues.

Tucker, Joseph D., Cedric H. Biena, and Rosanna W. Peeling. 2013. *Medscape.* http://www.medscape.com/viewarticle/777839. Accessed on March 30, 2017.
This article provides an introduction to the concept and practice of point-of-care procedures for the testing for a variety of STIs, along with a review of the current technology available in this field.

Tufel, Gary. 2016. "Sexually Transmitted Infections Present Diagnostic Challenges." *CLP.* http://www.clpmag.com/2016/07/ sexually-transmitted-infections-present-diagnostic-challenges/. Accessed on March 30, 2017.
The author offers this reminder that recognizing the presence of al STI can pose difficult problems for a health care worker. This article explains why that situation is the case and what that future prospects for diagnostic procedures are.

Vagianosa, Alanna. 2017. "Short Film Explores What It's Like to Find Out You Have an STI." *Huffington Post*. http://www. huffingtonpost.com/entry/short-film-explores-what-its-like-to-find-out-you-have-an-sti_us_58cff9fce4b0ec9d29ddaa56. Accessed on March 29, 2017.

> This web article discusses a new short film that illustrates what it is like to find out that one has an STI. A link to the film is provided on the web page.

Whitman, Hallie, and Stephanie Cajigal. 2016. "Timeline: 10 Years of the HPV Vaccine." *Medscape*. http://www.medscape. com/viewarticle/866964_4. Accessed on March 29, 2017.

> This excellent article reviews important steps in the approval, recommendations, and use of the HPV from (in spite of the title of the article) 1982 to 2016.

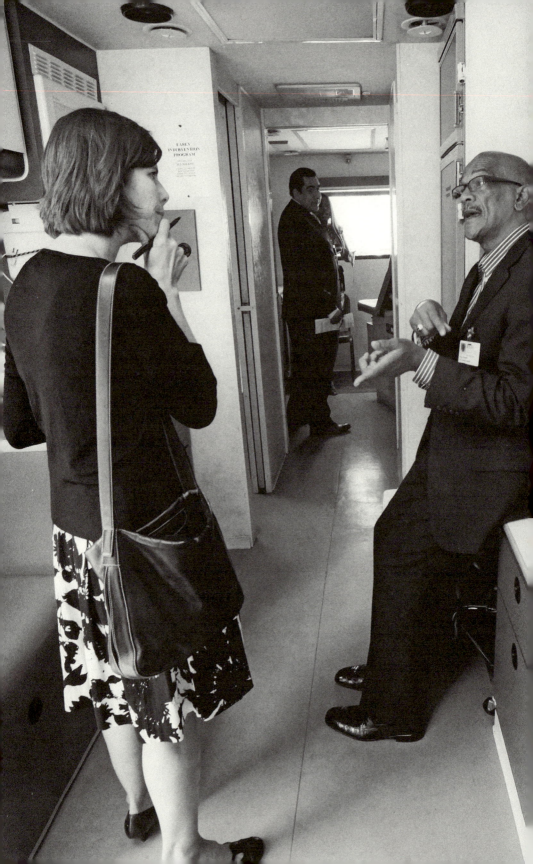

The story of sexually transmitted infections (STIs) among humans and other animals has a long and intriguing history. The following chronology lists some of the most important and interesting of the events that make up that history.

ca. 400 BCE   Greek physician Hippocrates describes a medical condition that he calls *strangury*, which many modern authorities regard as equivalent to the modern disease of gonorrhea. He also describes a condition in which painful, itchy lesions break out in the genital region, which he calls *herpein*, meaning "to creep." The condition is now known as *herpes*. Hippocrates also recognizes the characteristic yellowing of the skin characteristic of another sexually transmitted disease (STD), hepatitis.

30 CE   In his six-volume work *De Medicina*, Roman physician Aulus Cornelius Celsus describes a medical condition characterized by the presence of painful lesions that appear around the mouth. Later called *herpes labialis* by physician Herodotus, the condition is now known as *oral herpes*. A decade earlier, in 14 CE, Emperor Tiberius had banned kissing during public events in an effort to prevent the spread of oral herpes among the general public.

An HIV counselor explains to a visitor how a mobile testing center operates. The program provides young women in South Los Angeles with home-testing kits for sexually transmitted diseases. (AP Photo/Reed Saxon)

115 CE   Gaius Caecilius Pliny (Pliny the Younger) is one of many early physicians to take note of a medical condition characterized by a discharge of a milky fluid from the penis, almost certainly gonorrhea. Pliny calls the condition *profluvium genitalis viris*, "spillage from a man's penis."

130 CE   Roman physician Galen assigns the modern name of *gonorrhea* to the condition formerly called *strangury* by Hippocrates.

1162   The date often given as that of the first law concerning STIs, decreed by the Bishop of Winchester against houses of prostitution.

1343   Joanna I, queen of Both Sicilies, decrees that "if one [a prostitute] is found who has contracted a disease from coitus, she shall be separated from the rest and live apart."

1376   English surgeon, John Arderne, describes a medical condition that he calls *chaude-pisse* (literally, "hot piss"), characterized by a burning sensation that occurs during urination. The condition, he says, occurs among both men and women. Arderne's description is thought to be the first dependable description of gonorrhea in history.

1490s   The first recorded appearance of syphilis in Europe, thought by some authorities to have been brought to the continent by sailors returning from voyages to the New World, where it already existed. Perhaps the earliest account dates to 1493, when medical records from the English town of Shrewsbury mention a "fowle scabe and horrible sickness called the freanche pocks."

1493   Spanish physician Ruy Dias de Isla describes a disease that has appeared in Barcelona that was "previously unknown, unseen and undescribed," but that was present in sailors returning from Columbus' voyages to the New World. This report is one of a handful at that time now regarded as proof that syphilis arose from the Western Hemisphere, and not from the Old World.

1494   A syphilis epidemic breaks out when an army under King Charles VIII invades Naples, starting a war that is to last for four years. By the end of the war, the disease has begun to spread throughout Europe.

1530   Italian physician Girolamo Fracastoro suggests the name *syphilis* for the medical condition previously called "the great pox." The name comes from his poem, "Syphilis sive Morbus Gallicus" (Syphilis, or the French Disease"), about a shepherd name Syphilis who was cursed with the disease by the god Apollo.

1546   Fracastoro writes his famous book, "De contagione et contagiosis morbis," (*On Contagion and Contagious Diseases*) in which he argues against the existing theory of disease as an imbalance in body humors and suggests that disease can be transmitted by direct contact or indirect contact between two individuals and at a distance between two individuals.

1564   In his book, "De Morbo Gallico" (*The French Disease*), Italian anatomist Gabriele Falloppio provides the first recorded instructions for the use of a condom.

1694   English physician provides the first known description of herpes and invents the modern name for the disease.

1714   English physician Daniel Turner first describes an infection of oral herpes in terms that would be familiar today.

1736   French physician Jean Astruc provides the first clinical description of genital herpes.

ca. 1813   The joint efforts of English physicians Robert Willan and Thomas Bateman result in a recognition of various types of herpes. They define six types, a categorization no longer accepted. But they do clarify the relationship between oral and genital herpes.

1835   French bacteriologist Alfred François Donné discovers the causative agent for trichinosis, an organism he calls *Trichomonsis vaginalis*.

1858   American-born French physician Philippe Ricord definitively describes the difference between syphilis and gonorrhea. He further identifies the three stages of syphilis known today as the primary, secondary, and tertiary (or late) stages of the disease.

1860   French dermatologist Auguste Vidal de Cassis publishes one of the first comprehensive descriptions of congenital syphilis in his book "De La Syphilis Congenitale."

1870   Vidal de Cassis demonstrates that herpes can be transmitted by contact between two individuals.

1873   The U.S. Congress passes the Comstock Act, legislation that makes it illegal for anyone to send information about abortion or contraceptives through the U.S. mail. The act is later used to strike down a number of public health programs that, in addition to these two subjects, offer information, guidance, and services relating to the prevention and treatment of STIs. (*See*, for example, 1916.)

1879   German physician Albert Neisser discovers the bacterium that causes gonorrhea, an organism that is later named in his honor as *Neisseria gonorrhoeae*.

1885   German researcher A. Lurman describes an outbreak of serum hepatitis among dockworkers in Bremen, Germany. He demonstrates that the epidemic is caused by transmission of the infection among men who have been inoculated against smallpox.

1889   Italian dermatologist Augusto Ducrey discovers the causative agent of chancroid, a bacterium now called in his honor *Haemophilus ducreyi*.

1897   German chemist Arthur Eichengrün discovers the first dependable cure for gonorrhea, a compound called silver proteinate, with the trade name of Protargol (also known as Argyrol). The product is no longer used for the treatment of gonorrhea, but may be effective for use with a variety of inflammatory diseases, such as adenoiditis, pharyngitis, otitis media, conjunctivitis, ophthalmia, and rhinitis.

1905   German researchers Fritz Schaudinn and Erich Hoffmann identify the causative agent of syphilis, which they name

Spirochaeta pallida. The name is later changed to its modern form of *Treponema pallidum*. They are unable, however, to provide evidence that the microbe actually causes syphilis. (*See also* **1913**.)

1906   A team of three German researchers at the Robert Koch Institute for Infectious Diseases, August Wassermann, Julius Citron, and Albert Neisser, develop the first reliable test for syphilis, a test later name the Wassermann test.

1907   Czech medical researcher Stanislaus von Prowazek and German radiologist Ludwig Halberstädter discover the causative agent of trachoma and a number of related infectious diseases, a microbe now known as *Chlamydia trachomatis*.

1910   German researcher Paul Ehrlich and his Japanese colleague Sahachiro Hata discovered a compound that destroys the *T. pallidum* bacterium, providing the first successful modern treatment for syphilis. The compound is called arsphenamine and marketed under the trade name of Salvarsan.

1913   Japanese bacteriologist Hideyo Noguchi discovers the presence of the *T. pallidum* bacterium in the brain of patients with paresis, a condition commonly found in individuals with late-stage syphilis. The research provides definite evidence for the bacterium as the causative agent for syphilis.

1914   Ehrlich (1910) develops a more effective form of arsphenamine, later to be marketed under the trade name of Neosalvarsan.

The American Social Hygiene Association (ASHA) is formed in New York City through the merger of two earlier STI organizations, the American Federation for Sex Hygiene and the American Vigilance Association. ASHA later changes its name to the American Sexual Health Association.

The American Sexual Health Association is formed through the merger of the American Federation for Sex Hygiene and the American Vigilance Association.

1916   Margaret Sanger, Ethyl Byrne, and Fania Mindell open a clinic in the Brownsville district of New York City for the purpose of providing women of the region with accurate information about family planning (ways of avoiding pregnancy).

1917 The *American Journal of Syphilis* is founded. It is reimagined in 1934—and for only a single year—as the *American Journal of Syphilis and Neurology*.

Austrian physician Julius Wagner-Jauregg recommends the induction of malaria in patients with third-stage syphilis. The treatment is based on the fact that the condition can be cured or ameliorated by high temperatures, which can be produced by a malarial infection. Wagner-Jauregg is awarded the 1927 Nobel Prize in Physiology or Medicine for his discovery. The use of malaria was considered an acceptable risk for the treatment of late-stage syphilis because malaria could be cured with quinine.

1918 The U.S. Congress passes the Chamberlain-Kahn Act in an effort to stem the growing spread of syphilis in the United States. The proximate reason for the legislation was the large number of draftees for the U.S. military who were testing positive for syphilis. One provision of the act permitted law enforcement agencies to detain, examine, and quarantine any woman suspected of having and/or transmitting the disease, a specification that purportedly resulted in the detention of more than 30,000 women (almost exclusively sex workers). The bill also provides for the creation of a Division of Venereal Disease with the U.S. Public Health Service (PHS).

1921 Austrian physician Benjamin Lipschutz proves that genital herpes is transmitted by the transfer of fluid from an infected person to an uninfected person.

1923 The International Union against Sexually Transmitted Infections is founded in Paris with the objective of reducing the incidence of STIs throughout the world.

1927 Romanian physician Aurel Babe uses a platinum loop to collect cells from a woman's cervix to detect the presence of cancer. His work is less familiar than that of Greek physician

George Nicholas Papanicolaou, who makes a similar discovery a year later.

1928   Greek physician George Nicholas Papanicolaou develops a method for diagnosing the earliest stages of cervical cancer. The method later becomes more widely known as the Papanicolaou test (or more simply, the "Pap test").

In a now-famous example of serendipity in scientific studies, Sir Alexander Fleming discovers that a rare type of mold, *Penicillium notatum*, kills an array of disease-causing organisms, such as streptococcus, meningococcus, and the diphtheria bacillus. From that mold, he extracts a substance now known as penicillin, which proves to be the most powerful agent against syphilis and gonorrhea ever discovered. Penicillin is no longer the drug of choice for treating most types of STIs because most strains of those STIs have grown immune to the drug.

1930   The Neisserian Medical Society of Massachusetts is formed. It is the first medical society devoted specifically and exclusively the study and treatment of a single STI, gonorrhea. It is also the parent of a series of such organizations, such as the American Neisserian Medical Society, the American Venereal Disease Association, and today's American Sexually Transmitted Disease Association.

1932   The PHS, in conjunction with the Tuskegee Institute, founded in 1881 as the Tuskegee Normal School for Colored Teachers, initiates a study of syphilis in black males. The study is called the "Tuskegee Study of Untreated Syphilis in the Negro Male," and includes 600 black men, two-thirds of whom do have the disease and one-third who do not. The study is designed to determine the effectiveness of various types of treatments for the disease. It is carried out, however, without the knowledge of its subjects as to its true purpose and with no effort to actually treat individuals with syphilis. The experiment continues until 1972, when news begins to become generally available about its purpose and methods. The study is now widely regarded as one of the most immoral and unethical studies done in the United States on an uninformed group of individuals who had no opportunity to provide their informed consent to their participation in the research.

1934   The American Neisserian Medical Society is founded. It is the first American organization formed to deal specifically with any STI.

The Columbia Broadcasting System (CBS) warns Surgeon General Thomas Parran that he may not use the words "syphilis" or "gonorrhea" in a broadcast lecture on "medical economics." Parran then declines to proceed with the program.

1935   The PHS carries out the first National Health Survey, designed to collect statistical information on STIs. The data collected are intended to provide a basis for legislative efforts to prevent and treat syphilis, gonorrhea, and other STIs. (*See also* **1956**.)

1936   Connecticut becomes the first state to require syphilis testing in order to obtain a marriage license.

President Franklin D. Roosevelt appoints physician Thomas Parran as the country's sixth surgeon general. Parran is generally recognized as one of the most influential individual for promoting understanding of STIs among the American public.

1937   Surgeon General Thomas Parran publishes a book, *Shadow on the Land: Syphilis*, that outlines the threat posed by the large number of syphilis cases then extant in the country. The book stirs the interest and concern not only of the general public, but also of federal and state policy makers who are motivated to develop programs for dealing with the disease.

1938   The U.S. Congress passes the Venereal Disease Control Act of 1938, also known as the La Follette-Bulwinkle Act for its two sponsors in the Senate and the House. A primary provision of the act is provision of block grants to individual states to study and improve their programs related to STIs.

The Living Newspaper project produces a play called "Spirochete," dealing with issues surrounding syphilis. The play opens in Chicago, but soon travels also to other cities, including Boston, Cincinnati, Portland (Oregon), and Seattle. The Living Newspaper project deals with important social issues of the day through a stage performance. It was a part of the Federal Theater Project created by the Roosevelt administration toward the end of the Great Depression.

1941 The American Venereal Disease Association takes over management of the *American Journal of Syphilis* and renames it the *American Journal of Syphilis, Gonorrhea, and Venereal Diseases*. The journal is the parent of the modern-day journal, *Sexually Transmitted Diseases*.

1943 Convinced that it must do controlled research on the treatment of syphilis patients, the PHS begins an experiment with prisoners at the United States Penitentiary at Terre Haute, Indiana. The experiment lasts only ten months as researchers are unable to find an effective means of infecting subjects with the disease. The Terre Haute experiment does, however, serve as a model for a more ambitious research study of a similar nature in Guatemala in 1946. (*See also* **1946**.)

Greek physician George Nicholas Papanicolaou publishes a paper on his method for diagnosing cervical cancer discovered 15 years earlier. According to the most recent data available (2013), 69.4 percent of women over the age of 18 have had a Pap test (or "Pap smear") in the preceding three years. That number has dropped steadily, but slowly, over the 25-year period from 74.4 percent in 1987 to its 2013 rate.

1946 The PHS initiates an experiment in Guatemala in which unsuspecting individuals are intentionally inoculated with the causative agents of syphilis, gonorrhea, and chancroid in order to test possible treatment materials and regimens for the diseases. The experiment continues through 1948.

The National Communicable Disease Center (CDC) is established in Atlanta, Georgia, to conduct field investigations, offer training programs, and devise mechanisms for the control of communicable diseases. The CDC's name is later changed to the Center for Disease Control and then to the Centers for Disease Control and Prevention, but always retaining the same acronym.

1953 The U.S. Patent Office issues a patent to the Eli Lilly drug company for the production of erythromycin, the first powerful alternative to penicillin for the treatment of STIs.

1954 In an early attempt to develop a vaccine against syphilis, 62 prisoners at New York state's Sing Sing prison are inoculated with *T. pallidum* and then with the experimental vaccine. The vaccine fails to provide protection to the prisoners, who are then cured of the disease by the use of penicillin. In charge of the experiment is Dr. John C. Cutler, then acting chief of the venereal disease program in the U.S. Public Health Service. Cutler had also been involved in the experiments in Terre Haute (1943) and Guatemala (1946) in which nonconsenting individuals were intentionally infected with syphilis for the purpose of research on the disease.

1956 The U.S. Congress passes the National Health Survey Act of 1956, designed "to secure accurate and current statistical information on the amount, distribution, and effects of illness and disability in the United States and the services rendered for or because of such conditions." Syphilis and gonorrhea are included among the specific infectious diseases covered by the survey. The program continues to the present day, now under the name of the National Health Interview Survey.

1964 Mary Calderone, Wallace Fulton, William Genne, Lester Kirkendall, Harold Lief, and Clark Vincent create the Sexuality Information and Education Council of the United States (SIECUS) for the purpose of providing more complete and more accurate information about human sexuality for adults, adolescents, and children in the United States.

1969 The U.S. Food and Drug Administration licenses a vaccine for the prevention of hepatitis B, developed by American medical researchers Baruch Blumberg and Irving Millman.

The vaccine is the first such product to become available for the prevention of an STI, hepatitis B.

1970   The U.S. Congress passes an amendment to the Public Health Service of 1944, the Communicable Disease Control Amendments of 1970, providing funds for programs designed to control the spread of STIs in the United States. Similar amendments are passed in 1972 (the Communicable Disease Control Amendments of 1972) and 1976 (the Disease Control Amendments of 1976).

1972   The first news articles about the Tuskegee experiment appear. Before the end of the year, PHS has discontinued that experiment. (*See* **1932**.)

1974   In a now-classic paper in the field, "Cancer of the Cervix: A Sexually Transmitted Infection?," British epidemiologist Valerie Beral suggests that sexual activity may be a major cause for cervical cancer.

German virologist Harald zur Hausen discovers that the human papillomavirus (HPV) is a causative agent for cervical cancer, an achievement for which he is awarded a share of the 2008 Nobel Prize in Physiology or Medicine.

1975   American virologists Stephen M. Feinstone, Albert Kapikian, and Robert H. Purcell demonstrate that hepatitis A ("infectious hepatitis") is caused by a virus now known as the hepatitis A virus or, more commonly, HAV.

1977   The International Society for Sexually Transmitted Diseases Research is founded in Rotterdam for the purpose of encouraging research on STIs and to provide an avenue by which such researchers can share information with each other.

1981   The first cases of acquired immune deficiency syndrome (AIDS) are reported in the United States. A total of 234 men have died of the disease by the end of the year.

A group of concerned gay and nongay men meet in New York City to form an organization to gain funding and produce educational materials about the new disease appearing among gay men in the United States (AIDS). The group, which continues today, takes the name of Gay Men's Health Crisis.

A team of American, British, and French researchers report the discovery of a new organism responsible for the development of nongonococcal urethritis. The pathogen is also later hypothesized to be a cofactor in human immunodeficiency virus (HIV) infections.

1983 In response to the perceived need for an organization to carry out educational programs about and to fund research on the growing AIDS epidemic in the United States, a group of individuals meet in New York City to establish the AIDS Medical Foundation (AMF). Two years later, AMF merges with the National AIDS Research Foundation, a recently formed California corporation with roughly the same objectives as its own. The new entity is called the Foundation for AIDS Research, more commonly known by its acronym of amfAR.

French researcher Luc Montagnier and his colleagues discovered a possible causative agent for HIV infections, a virus they call the lymphadenopathy-associated virus.

A research team led by German virologist provides definitive evidence that HPV infections are related to, and almost certainly cause, at least some faction of all cervical cancer.

1984 San Francisco residents Martin Delaney and Joe Brewer found Project Inform, an organization designed to provide men and women infected with HIV with information about new drugs that were being studied for the treatment of AIDS.

1985 The U.S. Food and Drug Administration (FDA) announces a policy that permanently "defers" any man who has had sex with another man, even once, since 1977, from donating blood, regardless of the man's actual HIV status.

1987 By direction of the U.S. Congress, the U.S. Department of Health and Human Services announces that anyone testing positive for the HIV virus is ineligible for admission to the United States and that AIDS would be added to the list of "dangerous contagious diseases" that justified that ruling (Title VIII, Section 1182). The specific regulation reads that any alien "who is determined (in accordance with regulations prescribed by the Secretary of Health and Human Services) to have a communicable disease of public health significance, which shall include infection with the etiologic agent for acquired immune deficiency syndrome," is inadmissible to the United States.

1989 A team of researchers from CDC, National Institutes of Health, and the Chiron Corporation announce the discovery of a virus responsible for the diseases previously called non-A non-B hepatitis, now known as hepatitis C.

1990 The U.S. Congress passes the Ryan White Comprehensive AIDS Resources Emergency Act (Ryan White CARE Act). The act provided funding to extend and improve the availability of care for low-income, uninsured, and underinsured victims of AIDS and their families. The act is named for an Indiana teenager who contracted AIDS as the result of a blood transfer he received as treatment for his hemophilia. He died from the disease in 1990. The act is reauthorized in 1996, 2000, 2006, 2009, and 2013.

1992 The FDA revises its 1985 blood donation policy (*see* **1985**) to include commercial sex workers, those who inject illicit drugs, and certain individuals with other risk factors.

1993 The FDA announces its approval of the first female condom, the Reality Female Condom, a device shown to provide "highly effective protection" against the transmission of sexually related infections.

1994 The National Center for HIV, STD, and TB Prevention is created within the CDC to coordinate the agency's HIV prevention, STI prevention, and tuberculosis elimination programs.

1995 The FDA grants approval for the commercial production of the first hepatitis A vaccine, Havrix. Later in the same year, FDA approves the use of a second hepatitis A vaccine with the trade name of Vaqta.

The FDA approves the use of valacyclovir (Valtrex) for use in the treatment of herpes simplex viruses and varicella zoster virus infections.

1997 The National Coalition of STD Directors is formed for the purpose of coordinating efforts of state STD officials and promoting education about the nature, transmission, prevention, and treatment of STIs.

2003 Luc Montagnier and Robert Gallo publish a joint paper in the *New England Journal of Medicine* in which they agree on the contributions of each researcher to the discovery of the human immunodeficiency virus (HIV).

2006 The FDA grants approval for the production and sale of the first HPV vaccine, trade named Gardasil, in the United States.

2007 The World Health Organization announces that sufficient empirical evidence exists to confirm that HPV infections are responsible for a significant number of oropharyngeal (mouth and pharynx) cancers.

2008 In the case of *Rossiter v. Evans*, the Iowa Supreme Court rules in favor of the plaintiff, who became infected with HPV and developed genital warts as the result of a sexual encounter with Evans. The court awarded damages to Rossiter in the amount of $1.5 million in the case. The judgment was based in part on the decision of a lower court that the defendant's conduct "constituted a willful and wanton disregard for the rights or safety of another."

2009 President Barack Obama announces the discontinuation of a ban on the entry of HIV positive people to the United States from foreign countries. (*See also* **1987**.)

2010 The U.S. Congress passes the Affordable Care Act, which, along with many other provisions, significantly increases the prevention and treatment options available to individuals with an STI.

Wellesley College medical historian Susan M. Reverby discovers documents revealing actions of PHS researchers during the 1940s in Guatemala, in which subjects, without their understanding of the experiment or provided with a change to give their consent, were intentionally inoculated with *T. pallidum* in order to test possible treatments for syphilis.

2012 Mississippi becomes the last state to discontinue its requirement of a blood test for syphilis in order to obtain a marriage license.

The CDC reports that, according to the latest data available, the rate of STIs among Americans in the 50–80 years of age group has more than doubled over the preceding decades. The cause for this trend appears that seniors are taking fewer safer sex precautions than in the past.

2013 The American Sexually Transmitted Disease Association changes the name of its primary annual award from the Thomas Parran Award to the ASTDA Distinguished Career Award because of recently undiscovered and unethical research programs by the individual (Parran) for whom it was originally named.

The Ryan White Act of 1990 is reauthorized for the fifth time, with an annual budget for HIV/AIDS prevention and treatment programs set at about $2.3 billion. The program is the federal government's largest single mechanism for dealing exclusively and specifically with the nation's HIV/AIDS problem.

2014 National Network of STD Clinical Prevention Training Centers is created as a mechanism for increasing knowledge of health professionals and clinicians about STIs and related issues.

2015 The FDA announces a change in its 30-year-old policy on blood donation by men who have sex with men. The changes a lifetime deferral for such conations to a one-year deferral since the last sexual contact with another man.

A total of 842 citizens of Guatemala sue Johns Hopkins University for more than a billion dollars because of their role in a 1946 STI experiment in which university researchers participated. The case is thrown out of court by the presiding judge a year later.

2016　President Barack Obama orders the removal of three STIs from the list of infectious diseases for which an individual can be prohibited from entry to the United States. The three diseases are chancroid, granuloma inguinale, and lymphogranuloma venereum.

2017　In his proposed federal budget for FY 2018, President Donald Trump asks for a continuation of the Ryan White Act program for dealing with HIV/AIDS issues in the country. (*See also* **1990**.)

Glossary

Discussions of sexually transmitted diseases often involve terminology that is unfamiliar to the average person. In some cases, the terms are scientific or medical expressions used most commonly by professionals in the field. In other cases, the terms may be part of the everyday vernacular that some people may *think* they understand, but that actually have more precise meanings. This glossary defines some of those terms that have been used in this book, along with some terms that one may encounter in additional research on the topic.

abstinence   Voluntary decision by a person not to engage in sexual intercourse with another person.

acute   In medicine, an abrupt, often short-lived condition that may progress rapidly and require immediate attention.

alternative and complementary medicine   Methods for treating disease other than those used by conventional Western medicine. They include the use of herbs, acupuncture, massage, and traditional Chinese medicine.

anal intercourse   Sexual activity that involves the insertion of the penis into the anus.

antibiotic   A type of medication that is effective against bacterial infections, but that has no effect on viral infections.

antiviral   A type of medication that disables or kills a virus.

asymptomatic   Without signs or symptoms of an infection. A person may have been infected by a microorganism, but not yet show any outward indications of the presence of that agent within his or her body.

bacterial vaginosis   A condition caused by excessive bacterial growth within the vagina, resulting in a variety of STDs. Formerly known as nonspecific vaginitis.

bubo   A swelling of the nymph nodes, frequently a sign of some type of infection.

burden of disease   The impact of a given health problem in terms of its morbidity, mortality, economic cost, and other measures. *See also* **disability-adjusted life years** and **quality-adjusted life years**.

celibacy   The decision by a person not to engage in sexual relationships or sexual activities.

cervix   The narrow, neck-like passage at the lower end of the uterus.

chronic   A medical condition that tends to appear and develop slowly over a long period of time.

contagious   Capable of being transmitted from one organism to another organism, through either direct or indirect contact.

cryotherapy   A form of medical treatment that involves freezing a part of the body with liquid nitrogen. Cryotherapy is one method of treating genital warts.

dementia   A medical condition in which one loses one or more mental functions, such as memory or the ability to reason normally.

dental dam   A flexible plastic material that can be used to prevent transmission of a disease during oral, anal, or vaginal intercourse.

disability-adjusted life years (DALY)   An indication of the number of years lost as result of the spread of some particular disease. *See also* **burden of disease**.

dyspareunia   Painful sexual intercourse.

dysuria   Difficult or painful urination.

ectopic A condition that occurs in some part of the body other than its normal condition. An ectopic pregnancy, for example, is one that occurs someplace other than the uterus.

Expedited Partner Therapy (EPT) The practice of treating sex partners of patients diagnosed with chlamydia or gonorrhea by providing prescriptions or medications for the patient to take to his or her partner without the health care provider's first examining the partners.

immunity A condition in which an organism is protected against an infection or disease, generally because of antibodies that exist within that organism's body.

immunodeficiency A medical condition in which an organism's immune system does not function properly, resulting in a greatly increased risk for that organism of infections that, in some cases, can be fatal.

incidence In medical statistics, the number of new cases of a disease reported within a given population over a given time, such as one year.

latency The period of time following infection by a disease-causing agent and the appearance of signs and/or symptoms of that disease.

men who have sex with men A relatively new medical term to describe gay men, bisexuals, and any other men whose sexual activity includes relationships with other men.

morbidity The presence of disease in a body. Also, the rate of a disease within a defined population.

mortality Death. Also the death rate within a given population.

MSM *See* **men who have sex with men.**

nonspecific vaginitis *See* **bacterial vaginosis.**

oral intercourse Any form of sexual activity in which the mouth comes into contact with the male or female genital region.

pap smear A diagnostic test in which fluid from the endo-cervical canal is sampled for abnormal cells that may indicate the presence of a cancerous or precancerous condition.

papule A small-rounded bump on the skin usually resulting from some type of infection that may or may not be painful and/or itchy.

pathogenic Capable of causing a disease.

prevalence In medical statistics, the total number of indi-viduals who have a particular medical condition as of some date of record.

prognosis The likelihood of various possible outcomes of an infection or disease.

purulent Producing or capable of producing pus.

pustule A small pimple-like structure on the skin that con-tains pus.

quality-adjusted life years (QALY) An indication of the number of years lost as result of the spread of some particular disease. *See also* **burden of disease**.

remission The disappearance of the signs and symptoms of a disease that may or may not indicate that the disease has been cured.

reportable disease A disease that, because of its potential seriousness to public health, must be reported to a local, state, or federal health agency.

screening The process of testing for the presence of a disease, such as an STD, before any signs or symptoms of the disease are present. Screening is typically performed on individuals who are known or thought to be at risk as a way of increasing the efficacy of treating an infection before it develops to a more dangerous stage.

seroconversion That period of time during which a person's body develops enough antibodies to the presence of a caus-ative agent that they can be detected by some type of testing procedure.

sign In medicine, the indication of an abnormal health condition that can be detected by an outside observer. A high temperature, for example, is a sign because it can be measured by a thermometer.

surveillance The collection of data and statistics about the incidence and prevalence of a disease, with the goal of developing programs for the prevention and treatment of that disease.

symptom The indication of an abnormal health condition observed by the person experiencing that sensation, but not visible or otherwise detectable by another person. A headache is an example of a symptom.

topical agent A substance that is applied to the skin or some other surface.

urethritis Inflammation of the urethra.

vaginal discharge The release of a fluid from the glands of the vaginal wall.

vaginal intercourse Any form of sexual activity that involves insertion of the penis into the vagina.

abortion
AFY programs on, 162
Planned Parenthood
services, 66, 201
spontaneous, 148, 149
abstinence, 146, 155, 162,
180, 250, 256
"Abstinence-Only-
Until-Marriage
Programs: Ineffective,
Unethical, and Poor
Public Health" (AFY),
162–163
abstinence-only-
until-marriage
sex education
programs, 207
"Achieving the Millennium
Development Goals"
(AFY), 163
acquired immune deficiency
syndrome (AIDS)
ASHA publications
on, 164

epidemic, 167–168,
180, 187
vaccine for, 36, 40, 92–94,
167–168
See also human
immunodeficiency virus
(HIV)
ACT UP (AIDS Coalition to
Unleash Power), 187
acute epididymitis, 26
acute hepatitis, 96–97
acute juvenile rheumatoid
arthritis, 15, 84
Advocates for Youth (AFY),
161–163
Affordable Care Act of
2010, 66
African Americans. *See* Black/
African Americans
AFY (Advocates for Youth),
161–163
AIDS. *See* acquired immune
deficiency syndrome
(AIDS)

About the Author

David E. Newton holds an associate's degree in science from Grand Rapids (Michigan) Junior College, a BA in chemistry (with high distinction), an MA in education from the University of Michigan, and an EdD in science education from Harvard University. He is the author of more than 400 textbooks, encyclopedias, resource books, research manuals, laboratory manuals, trade books, and other educational materials. He taught mathematics, chemistry, and physical science in Grand Rapids, Michigan, for 13 years; was professor of chemistry and physics at Salem State College in Massachusetts for 15 years; and was adjunct professor in the College of Professional Studies at the University of San Francisco for 10 years.

The author's previous books for ABC CLIO include *Global Warming* (1993), *Gay and Lesbian Rights—A Resource Handbook* (1994, 2009), *The Ozone Dilemma* (1995), *Violence and the Mass Media* (1996), *Environmental Justice* (1996, 2009), *Encyclopedia of Cryptology* (1997), *Social Issues in Science and Technology: An Encyclopedia* (1999), *DNA Technology* (2009), *Sexual Health* (2010), *The Animal Experimentation Debate* (2013), *Marijuana* (2013), *World Energy Crisis* (2013), *Steroids and Doping in Sports* (2014), *GMO Food* (2014), *Science and Political Controversy* (2014), *Wind Energy* (2015), *Fracking* (2015), *Solar Energy* (2015), *Youth Substance Abuse* (2016), and *Global Water Crisis* (2016). His other recent books include *Physics: Oryx Frontiers of Science Series* (2000), *Sick!* (4 volumes) (2000), *Science, Technology, and Society: The Impact of Science in the 19th Century* (2 volumes; 2001), *Encyclopedia of*

Fire (2002), *Molecular Nanotechnology: Oryx Frontiers of Science Series* (2002), *Encyclopedia of Water* (2003), *Encyclopedia of Air* (2004), *The New Chemistry* (6 volumes; 2007), *Nuclear Power* (2005), *Stem Cell Research* (2006), *Latinos in the Sciences, Math, and Professions* (2007), and *DNA Evidence and Forensic Science* (2008). He has also been an updating and consulting editor on a number of books and reference works, including *Chemical Compounds* (2005), *Chemical Elements* (2006), *Encyclopedia of Endangered Species* (2006), *World of Mathematics* (2006), *World of Chemistry* (2006), *World of Health* (2006), *UXL Encyclopedia of Science* (2007), *Alternative Medicine* (2008), *Grzimek's Animal Life Encyclopedia* (2009), *Community Health* (2009), *Genetic Medicine* (2009), *The Gale Encyclopedia of Medicine* (2010–2011), *The Gale Encyclopedia of Alternative Medicine* (2013), *Discoveries in Modern Science: Exploration, Invention, and Technology* (2013–2014), and *Science in Context* (2013–2014).